THE FIRST-TIME FATHER'S HANDBOOK

DAD'S WEEKLY GUIDE TO EARLY FATHERHOOD AND
THE 9 MONTHS OF PREGNANCY

CAL PATER

CONTENTS

SPECIAL GIFT
JUST FOR YOU!

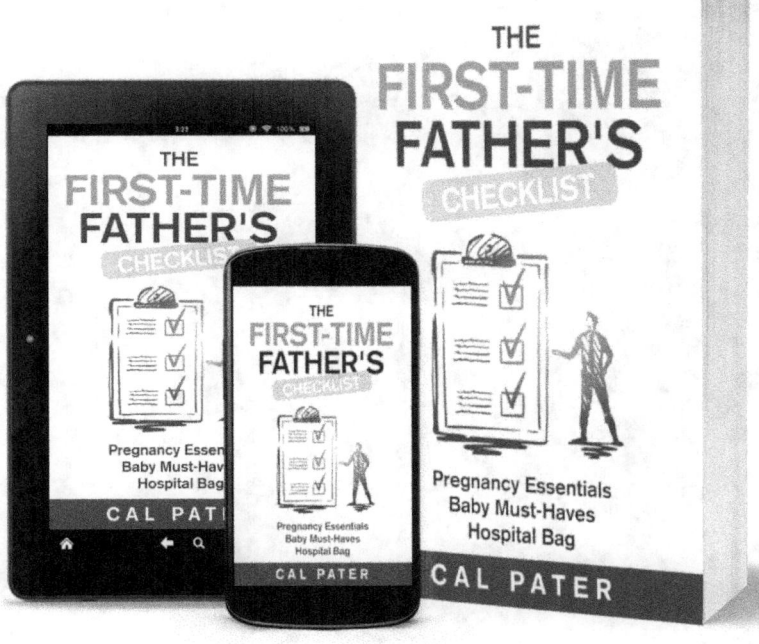

This Free Checklist has every item you need to make sure you go from dude to dad as smoothly as possible. Just visit the link.

WWW.FIRST-TIMEFATHER.COM

"Fathers, like mothers, are not born. Men grow into fathers and fathering is a very important stage in their development."

— DAVID GOTTESMAN

INTRODUCTION

"Your life will never be the same!" The words kept echoing in my head as I remembered the backyard barbecue when one of my buddies had announced that he and his wife were pregnant. We congratulated him in the only way we knew how—by teasing him. We kept reminding him of how his life would be completely different now, and I have to say, he took it like a champ.

At that point, though I had said it to my friend, I had no idea what those words meant. "Your life will never be the same." Honestly, I found it a bit weird when couples said *they* were pregnant. I mean, men don't get pregnant! That's plain and simple biology! Then why the fluff! Sure, becoming a father would come with a lot of responsibility, but that's only after the baby is born, right?

Wrong. As you may have guessed, I had no clue what was coming my way when *we* (me and my wife) decided to get pregnant. So yes, the journey from "My wife is pregnant." to "*We* are pregnant." wasn't an easy one. But here I am today, a proud dad of one and a to-be dad of another, and I wouldn't have it any other way!

When we first saw the two lines on the pregnancy test stick, we were over the moon. I was going to be a new dad after all! But once the excitement faded, panic quickly took over. Both of us were clueless as to what this would entail. Like anyone else, we wanted to make sure we did *everything* right. Not just right but perfect. So, we made quite a few trips to the bookstore during our first pregnancy. And at the end of each of those visits, my wife would come back with a tall pile of books about what to do and how to do it. On the other hand, I would be lucky if I found a flimsy pamphlet-sized magazine to let me know how to make my wife *comfortable* in this vulnerable time. I swear I even read a piece about how men are more likely to cheat when their wives are pregnant. Way to boost my confidence!

While I was happy to do all that I could to make my wife as comfortable as possible, I soon started feeling like I had no other role in this supposedly life-altering event. Why was no one talking about the father's role in the pregnancy? Or was that role so obvious that no one bothered to tell you about it? If it was, then how could I be missing out on such obvious expectations? What if I never figured it out even after the baby was born?! I was freaked out by these thoughts way too often.

That is the precise reason I want to reach out to you, an expectant father, and tell you all of what I have learned. And believe me, it's more than just making your partner comfortable. If you, like I did at the beginning of our pregnancy, assume that your role is to come in only when the baby comes out, you are in for a rude awakening. You don't suddenly become a father overnight. It's a gradual process. I am here to tell you that this process doesn't have to be difficult but it can be one of the most precious experiences of your life. The more involved you are in the pregnancy at the beginning, the easier you'll find it to transition into a dad's role when the baby comes into your world.

This book is designed to make this transition as fulfilling and effective as possible. But before we move on to the actual journey, let's first get a few things out of the way.

It's no secret that, like everything else around, father-hood has also evolved immensely. The challenges that new dads face today are widely different from the ones their older counterparts faced. Without addressing the ever-evolving role of a new dad, we would never be able to fully understand this sometimes overwhelming experience of taking on the complete responsibility for a life.

YOU ARE A DAD WHEN...

Think about it—what is it that makes you a parent? When do you stop being a dude and start feeling like a dad? It's difficult to pinpoint that exact moment, isn't it? Many parents remember it as the moment they held that tiny baby in their arms. Many others describe it as the moment they hold that positive pregnancy test in their hands. But the truth is, you need neither of these to become a parent.

Adoptive parents, for instance, might relate very well to the fact that you become a parent when you decide to be one. The thing about parenthood is that biology is of the least significance here. Whether or not you are carrying a baby, you are still just as emotionally pregnant as any other person physically carrying a baby. A lot of research points to the fact that adoptive fathers go through many of the same issues as biological fathers.

This book is for anyone who thinks of themselves as a father—biological, adoptive, accidental, stepfather, whichever it is. The idea is to let you know that you can get all the help you need during those nine months and a little after that as well. This is the reason why, wherever applicable, I have tried to bring in all of these perspectives to help you make sense of the emotional journey you are embarking upon.

FULFILLING THE EXPECTATIONS

Traditionally, society has placed high levels of emphasis on the experience of becoming a mother rather than becoming a father. Why so, you ask? A lot of factors may have contributed, including the evolutionary perspective that looked at men as protectors and women as nurturers. Though the biological basis for this distinction may stand, it's safe to say we have all come a long way from when one gender had to protect the other from the physical dangers encountered in daily living. And yet, even today, the majority of childbearing and rearing issues are somehow implicitly considered as women's concerns rather than that of a couple.

The good news is that things are changing and societal expectations are increasingly roping in fathers. Men today want to be as involved as possible, regardless of these expectations. Most men, once they get over their cluelessness, report wanting to do as much as they can to make this a smooth-sailing process. But the problem lies in that men have never been informed of how to navigate these (amniotic) waters. Since your sex-ed class, you have been taught how to avoid pregnancy but no one has yet bothered to tell you what to do when you don't wish to avoid it anymore. That's like expecting a baby to walk with a perfect graceful gait while it hasn't even learned to hold up its head.

Societal expectations are, however, not the only measure against which you gauge your performance as a dad. More crucial are the expectations that you have set for yourself. If you have ever caught yourself saying, "I would never be that kind of a dad!" then you know exactly what I am talking about. One of the major tasks of fatherhood that you'll face is to find the right balance between the kind of a dad people want you to be and the kind that you are.

Well, brace yourself because the roller-coaster is just beginning!

WHERE DOES THIS BOOK FIT IN?

The fact that you have picked up this book tells me you want to do it the right way right from the beginning.

This book aims to prepare you physically, emotionally, and financially for your first-ever pregnancy.

The book is structured to give you a month-by-month picture of how the pregnancy will look for all three of you—your partner, your baby, and yourself. Each chapter is further broken down into the week-by-week happenings. At each stage, I give you some tips that I have found to be the most valuable.

But I wish to emphasize the fact that this is not just about the physical but also the psychological preparation that goes into it. And that is why we begin our first chapter with the common concerns that new dads are most likely to face. It is only after we have cleared these that we move into the actual pregnancy process over the next several chapters.

However, that's not where the journey ends. Once you have brought your baby home, we discuss the top three priority concerns that are likely to have the most impact on your life as a new dad—finances, your changing relationship with your partner, and your self-care.

It's only when you have this holistic understanding of all the aspects involved that you can be fully prepared for what's coming your way. Actually, scratch that. You can never be fully prepared for the way that little kid is going to change you forever but what you can do is give it the best shot possible and hope that you find your way through it relatively unscathed.

And now that I have terrified you enough, it's time to dig in and dad-up!

1

CONGRATULATIONS, YOU'RE EXPECTING!

The missed period. The first is a series of events that are going to change you and your partner's life. While you can take many of the tests from the first day of the missed period, the accuracy of the result will be much higher if you take it about a week past the date.

Also, now would be the perfect time to let you know that if you are someone who feels distinctly uncomfortable talking about your partner's menstrual cycle, then you better get used to it. You'll need to have similar conversations quite a bit.

For now, let's get back to the discovery of pregnancy. It's only when the shock and excitement of this news fade off, that you will have the time to process it in practical, realistic terms. This is when the panic sets in with the what's, when's, and how's of the actual process. Well, I am here to tell you that you are not alone. I have yet to meet a father (or even a mother, for that matter) who thinks they are completely ready for the pregnancy, no matter how deliberate the decision to have kids might be.

Regardless of how many books you read, and how many people you consult, nothing and no one can prepare you for the ride you are about to take. But if that's the case, then what's the point of this book? To tell you the truth, this experience is just as universal as it is personal. By that, I mean that while you will have tremendously unique, idiosyncratic, and intimate experiences throughout this process, you will also find many things that you will share with first-time parents all over. That's why it is crucial to have this conversation. Conversations, especially about first-time father experiences, can be put on the back burner much more often.

This book aims to bring all those conversations and experiences back into focus. In this chapter, we deal with the common concerns that you are likely to face when that pregnancy test flashes two lines. While it may not give you a solution for every concern, it helps to know that you are not alone, that you can reach out and find a listening ear at least, if not a helping hand. Believe it or not, these conversations will help you manage your own expectations for the coming nine months.

FIRST THINGS FIRST FOR FIRST-TIME DADS

The night following the discovery that we were pregnant, I laid wide awake in my bed, my head overcrowded with what seemed like a million questions. I am pretty certain my wife laid awake too. But neither of us talked to each other about it for the fear that it would dampen the happy mood somehow. That was my first mistake—not telling my partner what was going on in my head. More on this later but for now it would suffice to say, there are some aspects you need to clarify with your partner as soon as possible. In this section, I outline the most crucial things you'd want to get out of the way before anything else.

The When

Now that you are pregnant, the first thing you'll want to know is the exact day the baby is coming or as it is often called the 'due date'. You might hear the abbreviation EDD being thrown around by the doctors. This is simply a fancy way of saying the estimated date of delivery. There are two ways this date can be calculated. The first method is where you are certain of the date the baby was conceived and the second is when you would take into consideration your partner's last period.

The pregnancy is considered to begin from the first day of your partner's last period. Thus, the due date is considered to be 280 days or 40 weeks after this day. If you know the exact date that you conceived you'll just add 266 days to this day and you'll have the due date.

If neither is known, the doctor might even ask your partner to get an ultrasound to estimate how far along you are. But while a lot of emphasis is placed upon determining the due date, you want to remember that only a small percentage of babies are actually delivered on the due date. Likely, the baby might just decide to pop out a little sooner or may even decide to sit back and relax, refusing to come out until later. Your doctor will be able to monitor the baby's progress to decide if intervention is needed or not.

The Where

At this point, you are aware of when the baby is coming and the general timeline that you have on your hands to figure things out physically as well as emotionally. It may seem like nine months is a lot of time but take it from me, these months will pass in the blink of an eye. This is why you need to figure out the basic details right from the beginning. While many of these questions will be determined by your financial situation to some extent, you still need as much clarity as possible on these, to say the least.

One of the first questions you will decide upon is where the delivery would take place—in a hospital or a home. Over the last few decades, there have been fluctuating shifts in the preference of birthing parents. For instance, the mid-2000s saw a sharp rise in the preference for home births. People preferred to bring their child into this world in a familiar place amid their family. The reasons for this preference are numerous ranging from lack of easy access to hospitals, religious beliefs, financial constraints to just plain dissatisfaction with the medical services.

The other option is, of course, the hospital. Research suggests that hospital births are much safer than planned home births. The technological sophistication that hospitals allow in terms of monitoring the baby or even inducing labor if necessary cannot be replicated in home births.

If you and your partner are torn between the two, birthing centers might be a fair compromise. These are privately owned and mostly free-standing buildings that give you all the comforts of a home while also giving you the benefit of an assisted delivery with registered nurses and other trained professionals. They also have obstetricians on their teams that can be called upon in cases of emergencies.

Remember that this decision will also take into account certain factors like whether you are pregnant with a single baby, whether your baby is in the appropriate head-first position at the time of delivery and whether you have what can be termed as a low-risk pregnancy. If any of these conditions are not met, a hospital birth is your best option. Regardless of where you choose to give birth, you need to consult a healthcare provider and discuss your options in detail.

And a pro tip—whatever the decision, your partner needs to get the bigger say, because after all, she is the one carrying the baby in her body for all those months!

The Who

Another important decision you'll take here is to find the right professional to help you through the process. This needs to be a qualified individual whose judgment you can trust. If you and your partner wish to go in for a hospital birth, here are a few tips that you need to go over when choosing the best Ob/Gyn:

1. Consider the insurance coverage: Having health insurance doesn't mean you are automatically covered for all the medical expenses you have. Make sure you read the fine print to understand what your insurance does and does not cover. You might come across the phrase "in-network" in the context of insurance coverage. This refers to the hospitals that are covered under your insurance. Going out of the network can lead to quickly piling bills. So, until and unless there are some special complications, staying in-network is usually recommended.

2. Your partner's medical history: If your partner has chronic conditions like diabetes or cardiac disease, you might want to look at hospitals that provide special care. Sometimes it is possible to convince insurance companies to cover these expenses even if these hospitals may not be covered because such perinatal care can significantly reduce the future healthcare costs for the mother as well as the baby.

3. Choose an appropriate hospital and doctor: When choosing a hospital, you need to check out the services that are most relevant to you. You don't need fancy amenities as much as hospitals that have a good neonatal intensive

care unit (NICU) in case of any emergency, for instance. You might also want to consider the prenatal education programs that they offer and also their postnatal care and lactation support.

You want to make sure that whichever healthcare provider you choose is on the same page as you when it comes to aspects like medicated or unmedicated deliveries, C-sections, and so on.

THE ANXIETY AFTER THE EXCITEMENT

I wouldn't be exaggerating if I said this is the part I find most new dads struggling with. I am not ashamed to admit that in the beginning, I felt completely helpless dealing with my own demons. I knew all there was to know and yet I desperately kept looking for one answer —how on earth am I going to manage this?

Let's be honest. Not all of us have had the most perfect childhoods with rainbows and roses. A lot of how you see yourself as a parent comes from the parents who raised you. "My dad was super-strict, so I am going to be the exact opposite!" "I grew up with no rules in the house, so I am going to raise my kids with proper discipline." You may even decide to pick up a thing or two from your parents' parenting styles that worked for you.

Whatever it is, understanding where these expectations come from is the most important. While becoming a parent is one of the most amazing experiences in life, it is also one of the most trying. There will undoubtedly be times when you'll wonder what you've gotten yourself into. Remember that these mixed feelings are normal and you need to consciously prevent yourself from going on a guilt trip.

The Self-Doubt

When you find out about the pregnancy it's quite likely that you might feel overpowered by doubt and anxiety. Research suggests that men tend to experience much higher levels of stress when they are expecting than otherwise. For me, "Am I capable of taking care of something that tiny?", "Will I ever be a good dad?", and many more such thoughts ran on a loop in my head.

Though we would love it, the decision to become a parent doesn't come with a manual. But the good news is since there is no perfect way to do it, there also isn't a "wrong" way to do it. And that means you can make a rulebook of your own. The idea is not to become the perfect dad, there is no such thing. The point is to do the best you can because well, that's about as much as anyone can do.

Yes, I know this new role is scary. I have walked in those shoes. But if there's one thing I've learned, it is to not set impossible goals for myself as a father. Remember the first day at your first-ever job? Remember how overwhelmed you were? But you stuck through it and you will stick through this as well.

Having said that, though, I strongly recommend that you don't brush these thoughts under the carpet. In your attempt to "man up" you will probably only end up piling things on. The best way through these is to talk about them to your partner. Remember that you and your partner are in this together and you can lean on each other whenever you need to.

The End of Freedom?

I remember a colleague saying a long time back, "A baby is a final nail in the coffin of freedom." We had all laughed then and raised a drink to one of our friends beginning their journey of parenthood. Though meant as a joke, I, for one, truly believed that to be the case. How could the responsibilities of fatherhood be compatible with the carefree freedom of the past life?

This assumption went a long way in making me miserable when my wife was carrying. I found myself getting irritable a little too often thinking that my doom was approaching nearer by the day. I could not have been more wrong. It was only much later when I held that tiny life in my arms that I realized that none of the carefree ventures mattered anymore. It was at that moment that I realized that spending time with my child would never be an obligation, but something that I loved to do, something that I would move mountains for.

That might seem like a lot of fluff, something right out of a poem even. No, I am not romanticizing the idea of being a father. It's not all beautiful metaphors, not at all. But the joy of fatherhood is a personal experience that no metaphor can do justice to.

Having said that though, it helps to remind yourself now and again that being a father is a part of your identity. A big part, sure, but a part nonetheless. Becoming a father does not mean you have to give up the rest of your life completely. Yes, things will be different and the pregnancy may seem to be all of your life for a while and it will be. But as you and your partner get better with managing it, you both will find yourselves making a lot more room for other things that you care about, be it your social life, your hobbies, or even just a small amount of time for yourself. We talk more about this in the last chapter but for now, remember that embracing fatherhood will only add the dad layer to your cool personality.

Finances and the evolving relationship with your partner might be the other major concerns that we discuss in detail a little later in this book. But for now, it's time to get started with the pregnancy process.

2

THE FIRST MONTH

Your little swimmers have scored a victory and have fertilized your partner's egg. Though I say this in a brief sentence, this is anything but a simple journey for your sperm cells. Through the cervix which is an opening to your partner's womb, these tiny sperm cells reach the fallopian tubes where they meet the egg. This whole distance is about a thousand times the length of an average sperm. If your sperm can overcome all those obstacles to create a baby, then you can overcome the difficulties of raising that baby too!

SHARING THE JOY

As mentioned, it is often difficult to know exactly when you and your partner conceived but an estimate is usually made by using the first day of your partner's last period. It can be very tempting to share this joy with your loved ones as soon as you find out. But reign in your excitement there for a while! It's best not to share this news with too many people until your first trimester is over. This is because before this, the pregnancy is quite vulnerable and the chances of miscarriage are quite high. If God forbid a mishap occurs, going back and giving people the explanations over and over again can be quite traumatic in itself.

The first three months is the time that you can share the joy of parenthood among yourselves, unbeknownst to anyone else, quite like keeping a secret. Remember that during this time your life may hardly feel any different but your partner's body is surely going through an upheaval trying to accommodate a new life within it.

She will be required to cut out certain habits like the intake of coffee and alcohol. As a gesture of solidarity, you should stop taking them too. This might seem like a silly thing. "What good would it do to give up *my* morning coffee?" you may ask. Well, this will tell her that you are in this with her, that you are walking the talk, and that in itself is going to be massive psychological support for your partner.

THE WEEK-BY-WEEK PROGRESS

Now that you have sufficiently prepared for the pregnancy it's time to get to the nitty-gritty technical details. From here on out, I shall help you through each week of your pregnancy in the following sections:

- The baby's progress
- Your partner's experience
- What you can do

Let's dig in then, shall we?

Week 1

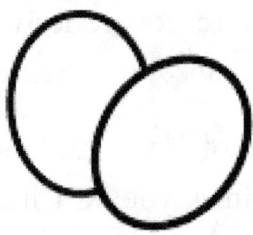

This is before you actually conceive. This is the preparatory phase before the baby comes in. This can be slightly confusing when tracking the pregnancy because in this week, technically there is no baby. But this is essentially because tracking periods is far easier than tracking ovulation, with the former showing more explicit physical signs than the latter.

In this week, your partner's body is gearing up for ovulation and subsequent pregnancy. This is a great time for your partner to start taking folic acid supplements. Folic acid or folate as it is known sometimes has proven to be highly beneficial in protecting the baby against neural tube defects like the underdevelopment of the spine (spina bifida) or underdevelopment of the brain (anencephaly). Note that these birth defects happen quite early in the pregnancy and thus Centers for Disease Control and Prevention (CDC) recommends your partner start taking 400 micrograms of folic acid even before you conceive. These are often said to lower your chances of miscarriage as well.

Folic acid is a type of B vitamin and helps in making new cells. Many times you will hear folate and folic acid used interchangeably but remember that they are a little different. Folate is a general term for B vitamin and is found in plenty in green leafy vegetables, asparagus, etc. On the other hand, folic acid is a man-made variant of folate and can be found in some fortified foods like rice, pasta, etc.

Week 2

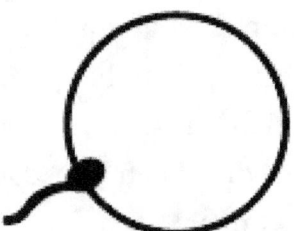

Much like the first week, in week two, there isn't a baby or a pregnancy at all. But your partner's body is all set for it as she is ovulating. The uterus is getting cozier and cozier with the lining becoming thicker in the anticipation of an egg fertilized by your champion sperms.

Your partner would start ovulating or releasing the egg from her ovary, by the end of the week. The cervical mucus can keep your sperm alive for up to five days. So, having sex a couple of days before the ovulation begins can get your little soldiers in position and ready for action when the egg comes down. Alternatively, you can have sex every other day while ovulation is in progress. With your partner's sex drive raging during this time, she would be up for it too.

Sex when trying to conceive is not the same as regular casual sex. As you can guess from the calculations above, it is much less spontaneous and may even feel quite mechanical. It's because of this that you might want to try "dating" your partner all over again. Though conception sex may be quite goal-oriented, it doesn't have to feel like a task. Go ahead and have some fun with it as you did when you dated your partner. Ask her out for dinner, exchange some steamy text messages, or gift her something that will spice up the whole process.

Note, however, that when trying to conceive, oral sex is out of bounds. The enzymes in saliva can get your little dudes pretty messed up. While the research in this area seems a little conflicted, why take chances?! Also, try to keep away from low-quality lubricants, hot tubs, and even electric blankets. Yup, now you know what I meant when I said sex to get pregnant is not the same as sex otherwise.

But despite doing all of the things, you may not conceive in the first go. It's important to stick to that schedule and keep at it. If, however, after persistent effort, you don't see results, then it might be time to consult a doctor. The doctor would then investigate the reasons why it hasn't yet worked out and may prescribe medication to increase those chances. If these meds work, conception will come at the small price of intense mood swings for your partner. These are likely a result of hormonal fluctuations due to the medication.

If, however, these meds do not work then you may have to brace yourself for the idea of an infertility clinic. "Doing it in a cup" is just as bad as it sounds but it's necessary to check if there are any concerns with the sperm. Your partner will also undergo some tests to determine if her uterine environment is conducive for pregnancy. This can create major stress and pressure to get the desired result as soon as possible. Whatever comes out of these embarrassing trips to these clinics, know that your partner has it a tad worse than you. Therefore, it's more crucial than ever that you stand by each other, firm and strong.

Week 3

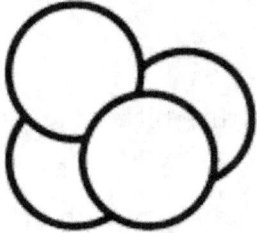 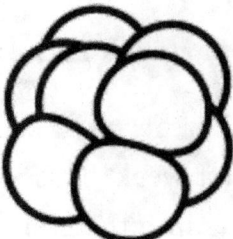

After all the sweat and semen, the part you have been waiting for is finally here. Your seed has fertilized the released egg and the resulting zygote is now traveling to the uterus. It is now building up into a ball of cells called the blastocyst which will later become the fetus and eventually the baby.

Your Baby's Growth

Believe it or not, at this point, your baby is the size of a head of a pin. The baby is growing at a fast pace as the cells divide and multiply in number. Around day five after fertilization, the blastocyst is now preparing to attach to the uterine wall. It is during this time that the single blastocyst can turn into multiple blastocysts resulting in multiple births. This is in the case of identical twins. But in the case of fraternal twins, rather than one single egg splitting up, two separate eggs become fertilized by two sperm cells. This is not very different from two separate pregnancies, only that your partner's ovaries have released two eggs instead of one.

Your Partner's Experience

Your partner may experience a tiny bit of bleeding in the first week. This is usually because the blastocyst is digging into the uterine wall in an attempt to attach to it. While doctors believe this is normal, not all women experience this.

Another thing you should be looking out for is your partner's mood swings. While your partner's body may not be changing on the outside, it is going through a lot of changes internally and that includes major hormonal fluctuations. An emotional roller-coaster awaits her and you have the front seat in there too.

What You Can Do

This is the perfect time for you to start making some healthy lifestyle choices. Whether it's working out together or simply going for a walk, it is great to show your partner that you care and are with her in this. Use caution when engaging in physical activities because you don't want your partner to strain herself too much. It's best to consult your doctor before making it a part of your routine.

It's also the best time to chuck those unhealthy eating habits and those takeouts and start shopping for groceries to cook your meals. These trips to the grocery store might just earn you some brownie points which will surely come in handy later.

Week 4

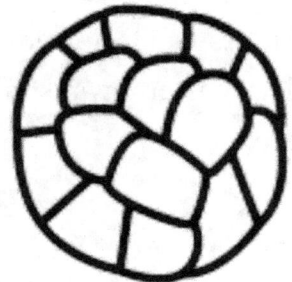 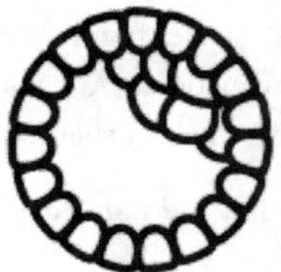

The baby is going to be in your partner's womb for a long time, it might as well get comfortable in there. During this week that's exactly what it's doing. During this time, it might be tough to distinguish early symptoms of pregnancy from the usual premenstrual experience.

Your Baby's Growth

The blastocyst is on a roll and is growing at a pretty fast pace. Some of these cells will turn into the embryo while others will take over the function of nourishing the embryo. This latter group of cells will start forming connections with the mother's blood supply from where it will derive nutrition for the baby. The former group, on the other hand, will continue to divide and specialize into three distinct layers.

- The top layer is like the neural headquarters which will later develop into structures like the brain, neural tube, nerves, and so on.
- The middle layer takes care of the circulatory mechanism, later developing into the heart, veins, and arteries.
- The last layer is for the other essential functions and later develops into lungs, intestines, urinary system, etc. But for now, it will be connected to the placenta which will take care of the nutrition and excretion functions for the baby.

When we talk about rapid development, it might give you a misleading impression about the baby's proportions. The truth is the embryo in no way resembles a baby at this point. Can you believe that right now the baby is only 0.04 inches long? That's right about the size of a poppy seed. Insignificant as that may sound, remember that it has made the journey from being the size of the head of a pin to poppy seed and that is quite the journey. What's more is that even though it might sound impossible, that poppy seed of a baby carries the genetic code for important characteristics like sex, eye color, hair type, and so on.

Another crucial development is the formation of the amniotic sac filled with amniotic fluid. This is where your baby will float nonchalantly for the next several months, protected from the traumas of daily living like temperature fluctuations or sudden jerks. This is when the bunch of cells is officially termed an embryo.

Your Partner's Experience

Even though it's early in the pregnancy, the hormonal changes in your partner's body are well on their way. The human chorionic gonadotropin (hcG) hormone levels are going to be extremely crucial around this time. The level of this hormone is what indicates pregnancy when your partner pees on that ever-important stick. HcG levels are seen to keep increasing until later in the pregnancy and this makes for a bunch of uneasy pregnancy experiences like frequent urination, exhaustion, tenderness of the breasts, food cravings, or aversions. But remember that these are still very similar to your partner's oncoming period woes. So, you both wouldn't know unless you take that test.

Another thing about pregnancy tests is that they don't give you a numerical value of the amount of hcG. For that, your partner will just need to go in for an old-school blood test. Higher hcG levels are also associated with multiple births. While it's way too early for an ultrasound, your healthcare provider might just be able to pick up on your partner's off-the-charts hcG levels to predict that twins (or more) might be on the way.

What You Can Do

The roller-coaster we mentioned earlier is just about to start and it's natural for you as well as your partner to be on edge. While the healthy lifestyle choices will continue, understand that this is not just an emotional experience for your partner but very much a biological one too. She might be experiencing these edgy emotions without even realizing what's causing them. And add to that the anxiety of knowing for sure whether she is pregnant or not doesn't make things any easier.

You might do well to distract her with activities that only the two of you undertake like going for walks or staying under the sheets watching a movie in bed or whatever it is that she seems up for. This does not mean you smother her with your care. Make sure she has enough time for herself too. Draw her a nice, relaxing bubble bath with the fancy bath salts. If you are like me, someone who had no idea about these things, looking things up on the internet might be a good place to start.

Take help from the ladies in your family and your friend circle to understand what you can do that might be comforting for your partner. Remember the gestures don't have to be grand. Even small actions like leaving each other surprise notes on the dresser or getting flowers delivered to her workplace might work like magic.

But most importantly, take this time to talk about both your feelings. A strong bond like that can go a long way in helping you and your partner through the difficult and overwhelming lows of this whole process.

So there it is! One down, eight more to go. You can be sure that it only gets more complicated from here, at least for a while until you settle in with the idea that you are going to be a new parent. The anxiety usually levels off around the middle of the pregnancy only to rise towards the end when the baby is actually about to come out. But hold your horses there before you start hyperventilating! Let's take this one month at a time, shall we? Onto the next month then, soldier!

3

THE SECOND MONTH

The peeing stick has spoken and you have been crowned dad to be and your partner mom to be. By this time, your anxiety over whether or not you're pregnant has likely turned into a panic over whether or not you'll be the kind of a parent that forgets their baby at Walmart. The next few months and your involvement in your partner's pregnancy will determine a lot of what your parenting journey will look like for the rest of your life.

Pregnancy tracking can be slightly tricky. Pregnancy is considered to be around 40 weeks which would technically be ten months. In medical terms, this would be the second month of the pregnancy, because the first month already began with your partner's last period. But many couples may not even be aware before this month arrives, as there are no explicit outward signs of the internal pregnancy.

THE WEEK-BY-WEEK PROGRESS

This is an exciting time for you as well as your partner but it can also be the most trying. Remember that the hormones are still raging in your partner's body and that can be truly difficult to cope with. It is only when you hold her hand through this time (sometimes physically and other times metaphorically), will you be able to defeat the beast of negativity and come out of this unscathed.

Week 5

Week five is a big week for all changes kicking in. Those internal affairs in your partners' body are now showing external signs too. At this point, you might find that your partner has a lot of reactions that neither of you really understand. Remember that this is the twisted work of those unpredictable hormones.

Your Baby's Growth

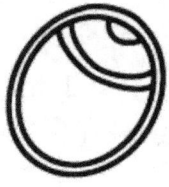 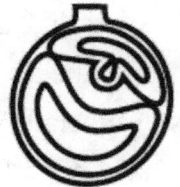 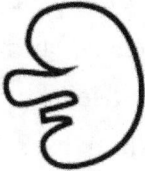

This week the weird ball of cells starts looking less like a blob and more like a tadpole. I know, I know! Blob? Tadpole? That's not what you signed up for. The stork version from your childhood was so much simpler, wasn't it? Well, this is the real world where storks have better things to do than deliver crying human babies. And your baby is getting there, slow and steady. From the poppy seed, it is now almost the size of a tiny lemon seed.

Remember the three layers we discussed last week? They are differentiating more and more now giving rise to specific human-like organs. The head of the tadpole-like structure remains the most noticeable part and it is going to stay that way for quite some time to come. But the embryo also has limb buds which will eventually grow into arms and legs.

Your Partner's Experience

The mother is still far from showing any external signs of pregnancy. But the signs like fatigue, tenderness of breasts, and nausea continue to get more and more intense. The tiredness especially becomes particularly visible as she might have to take more frequent pit stops even when climbing one flight of stairs.

Also, as the pregnancy continues to grow and press against her bladder, your partner's need to pee will only get more frequent. This can be frustrating as well as embarrassing for the mother, especially if she is in a professional set-up where her actions are being noticed by acquaintances.

What You Can Do

The best thing you can do at this point is to be mindful that regardless of whether or not her body has started showing explicit signs, she is literally housing a growing person within her body. That has to count as a 24x7 job. All those times that your mother sent you on a guilt trip saying she took care of you for nine months, well, that wasn't false.

At a time like this, you need to take charge. Make sure you take the initiative to make the grocery list, to remind her to take the supplements, to schedule the doctor's appointments, to tidy up the house, and whatever else there might be to do.

Also, don't forget to consider those bathroom breaks whenever you plan something special for her. Whether it's a candle-light dinner, a movie, or just a romantic long drive, your partner will probably need to go, more than once (or maybe multiple times).

Week 6

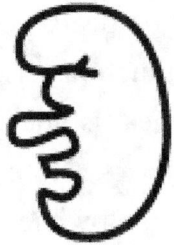

Week six is most likely the time that you have your first scheduled appointment with the healthcare provider. The uncomfortable pelvic test as well as the urine and blood screening may be your partner's first taste of the medical testing procedures to come over the next few months.

Your Baby's Growth

This week the fetus is on a roll and is making significant strides in terms of the development of human features. Your baby is now developing a face. All that tissue around its head will slowly transform into cheeks, chin, forehead, and jaw. The beginnings of eyes, nose, and ears are also visible by the end of this week.

Another organ that has a massive role to play in the baby's survival is the heart which is pumping faster every day. The expected heart rate around this time is somewhere around 110 beats per minute. Remember that this heart rate is much faster, almost double that of adults. A strong heartbeat is one of the signs that pregnancy is on the right track. Note that even though the heart is getting stronger by the day, this week might still be a tad early to hear it with an ultrasound but it sure isn't too far away. Though the heart is the star organ of this week, the kidneys, liver, and lungs are also building up their capacity in the background.

Your Partner's Experience

Week six can get very ugly for your partner very fast as ever-growing nausea becomes full-blown "morning sickness" which may not be limited to the mornings at all. Heartburn is going to kick in and your partner will be living with it until the end of the pregnancy. Your partner's diet will be a major factor here as she loses appetite for some food items and craves some peculiar other ones.

But the dark cloud of morning sickness has a silver lining of the "pregnancy glow". That means that your partner's hormones are getting her body in the best and strongest possible state to nurture that baby. Her hair might get thicker as the hormones prevent hair loss and her nails may become stronger too. Her breasts might also become larger due to these hormones. And last but not least, the curse of frequent urination continues to hover upon you both as a moth hovers around a flame.

What You Can Do

The most important thing you need to help your partner with this week is the preparation for the doctor's appointment. Prepare an elaborate list of questions to understand the process and also to get your Dos and Don'ts straight. Make sure to take an extensive look at both of your medical histories. Remember that pregnancy months are extraordinary times that require extraordinary measures. So, all those things that seem pretty okay for use and consumption otherwise may need your doctor's approval during pregnancy. That is why you must get everything clarified no matter how small or silly it may seem. It's always better to err on the side of seeming stupid than staying ignorant.

Another aspect where your partner will require your support is to motivate her to exercise. Now don't get too excited and act like you're Mickey training Rocky but getting those steps in with her might just do the trick.

You'll also need to watch out for any overwhelming emotions. Apart from her hormones running top gear, the physical restrictions she may feel due to the pregnancy might be just as overwhelming. Talk about the feelings and fears. The only way through it is together.

Week 7

This is the time that your tadpole starts transforming into a human baby. Well, it's not there yet completely, though the beginnings are unmissable. You might even call this the hands and feet week.

Your Baby's Growth

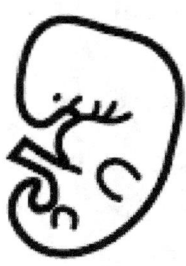

Been worried about that little tail on your baby? No need to worry anymore! That tail is getting smaller and will be gone soon. But that is hardly the highlight of this week. The baby is developing a skeletal structure but it's made of cartilage, soft and pliable. The buds that we saw on the embryo are now developing into legit hands and legs which are still flipper-like and tiny but they are closer to human hands than they have ever been.

This is also the time when the baby's heartbeat is stronger than before and it might even be ready to be heard over an ultrasound. This is one of the most exciting milestones you will cross as parents. As tiny as it might be, the baby is still almost 10,000 times bigger than the fertilized egg on the day of conception. As of now, it is almost the size of a blueberry. Though we are addressing it as a baby, keep in mind that it is still an embryo.

The head, which is the largest part in this week, houses the brain which is growing at a spectacular speed of almost a hundred cells per minute. The placenta which took its rudimentary shape somewhere during the fourth week is now developing a more and more complex structure preparing itself for a complete takeover of the baby's nutrition function in the coming few weeks.

Your Partner's Experience

If there is ever a secret superhero with a tremendous smelling capacity, your partner in the seventh week will without a doubt be a top contender. This is when her sensitivity to the slightest of smells will kick in. Combine that with the aversion to certain meats, dairy products, or other food items and it will be a task for her to not throw up every waking moment of the day, if she can get any sleep that is.

The uterus is now almost double its original size. But that's not all that's growing—your partner's breasts are also growing. But hey that might not always be good news because they may also feel tender and sore.

What You Can Do

A major task you'll take on at this point is cooking. Because of her sensitivity and aversions to certain foods and smells, you will have to be Captain Cook in your household for a while. Also, try asking her which fragrances she finds to be pleasant and use those in the form of air fresheners.

When it comes to physical activity while exercise is quite desirable, make sure she doesn't overdo it. It is crucial to take the doctor's opinion on what might and might not be good for the baby. For instance, the doctor might advise your partner not to engage in exercises that might result in a jerk to the abdomen area.

Medically, the coming few weeks might also be a good time to screen the embryo for any chromosomal concerns that might endanger the pregnancy. Make sure you ask your doctor about the same.

Week 8

This week, your baby is making the journey from being a blueberry to a raspberry. Quite the fruit salad you have on your plate there buddy! But the size is increasing and that's all that matters. The tail is completely gone (phew, thank god for that!) and from a tadpole just a few days back, the embryo looks like a legit human baby. The proportions of the body parts are still way off but the rapid changes are clearly visible.

Your Baby's Growth

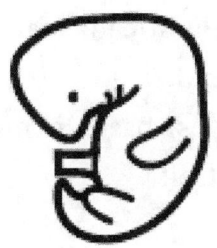

The baby's heart is beating at a crazy speed, more than almost twice the speed of the adult heart. But don't panic, this is completely normal for now. Remember those flipper-like limbs from the last week? They are now looking more distinct. You can make out the fingers and toes, though they're still webbed. The eyelids are also taking shape.

The baby's lungs are taking shape as the bronchial tubes branch out in the chest region. The neural network is also getting stronger and stronger as nerves spread throughout the baby's body. Note that now these nerves are not only creating connections among themselves but are connecting to the organs, the muscles, and the tissues too. This is setting up a foundation of a tremendously effective network that will fire extremely efficiently to carry the neural impulses.

Another interesting thing the embryo is doing this week is that it's moving around subtly. The movements are so negligible that your partner won't even feel them at this point. But insignificant as it may seem, note how the baby is slowly and steadily picking up on all adult functions in their most basic forms and that has to be quite significant in itself.

Your Partner's Experience

As the weeks pass by, your partner's discomfort is only going to get worse, physically as well emotionally. The pregnancy is still not showing on her waistline but the internal uterine enlargement can lead to some very unpleasant stomach soreness and tenderness.

All those symptoms like aversions, heightened sense of smell, and frequent need to pee are likely to be still going strong. But the aspect that's causing even more chaos in your partner's head is most likely the emotional mood swings resulting from the tumultuous hormones. This will cause a serious drain on her energy both physically and mentally. Low fatigue is quite a common symptom at this point on the curve.

Your partner may even experience occasional white discharge. Again this is common due to the increased quantities of estrogen in the body. But your partner needs to be mindful of the color of such discharge because any other color apart from white may just indicate some infection and require medical attention.

What You Can Do

If it hasn't become clear to you yet, it's high time you wake up and smell the beans—your partner is the rock-star here! She is the one experiencing all the changes first-hand. But you are like the backstage guy who does the soundcheck, the lighting, and basically everything else that lets the rockstar shine through.

You may not be able to help with everything but if you can pick up on the tiny things that you can do, that would be the best thing you'll do. So, make sure you stay patient through her mood swings, sometimes distract her with fun little things like board games or a little rock-n-roll karaoke, and other times help her talk through her feelings. Do this even when she flares up over little things or takes things too personally or goes in circles repeating the seemingly irrelevant things on a loop.

As this week draws to a close, celebrate getting through the second month alive and well, with a treat that your partner enjoys and won't hurl out even before it reaches her stomach. Yes, with this you have successfully gotten through the second month of your pregnancy. The first-trimester milestone is drawing closer every day.

4

THE THIRD MONTH

Two down, seven to go, and onto the third! Congratulations you have survived the first two months! Go ahead, celebrate with a cold beer! Enhhhh! That was a test my friend and if you fantasized about reaching out for that chilled can, rein in that rookie mistake! But drinks aside, celebrations are surely in order because you have survived two-thirds of the most crucial periods in your pregnancy.

What can I say here that hasn't been said about the first trimester? Well, it is the time when your baby is developing the most crucial functions necessary for survival. Moreover, you are quite close to clearing out of the danger zone of miscarriages and can soon share your good news with the loved ones that you have been itching to tell. A little more on that later but for now let's look at the week-wise development.

THE WEEK-BY-WEEK PROGRESS

For some, this can be an anxious time, with your partner having major difficulties keeping the food down. While these difficulties vary widely in severity, weight should definitely be on your watchlist. Weight loss due to excessive puking is quite the possibility and you'll likely have to find tailor-made solutions to this problem.

Week 9

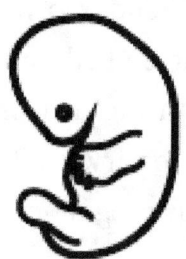

During this week you may not find major new changes happening but the embryo is only building upon its previous developments. The heartbeat is as strong as ever and the joint movements are more pronounced. There is still a long time to go before the mother will be able to feel this but the embryo is becoming more and more lively. A handheld Doppler ultrasound can detect multiple embryos and tell you if you are carrying multiples.

Your Baby's Growth

The embryo is around an inch long which is more or less the size of an olive. The embryo has come a long way from when it only had holes for eyes, ears, and nose. Now, these are much more prominent and can be seen as distinct features. The embryo is starting to look a lot like a person now.

Your Partner's Experience

Your partner's morning sickness is going to get much worse before it gets better. Experimenting with beverages like ginger tea can give her a lot of relief. Many women who experience horrible morning sickness also experience secondary discomforts like for instance, soreness in the throat, dehydration, etc. due to continuous puking. Ice chips can help relieve this soreness while also hydrating her body.

It is also very likely that she'll be irritable and refuse to take anything you give her. Be patient with her. Consider this as training to be a new daddy because believe it or not your baby, no matter how much you love it, will test you to your limits.

As the baby is growing within her, it's also demanding more nutrition. This can be especially difficult as she feels hungry and yet may find eating to be associated with the certainty of hurling afterward. But note that not all women experience this. While most of them experience nausea, only about half experience vomiting that's manageable to a great degree and only a tiny percentage of women experience the extremely severe symptoms. If your partner is among those unfortunate few then it's best to discuss this with your doctor because the constant puking also impacts the vitamins and the folic acid she is taking.

It is also advisable to be aware of the possible conditions that may arise as the pregnancy progresses. Many women experience gestational diabetes, gestational kidney stones, and many such conditions which are triggered by massive hormonal changes. Talking to your doctor can help you prepare for the necessary steps.

All the other symptoms like exhaustion, mood swings, and frequent urination are going to get worse. And here you were thinking that last week is as bad as it gets! Rookie mistake!

What You Can Do

Be there for her. She is most certainly going through a lot more than she is letting on. With so much going on, she might forget things like asking the healthcare provider the necessary questions or taking her vitamins on time. You being there for her through this and taking on the tasks she misses out on, will give her the confidence that you have her back.

You also need to start paying closer attention to what she is eating. Make sure despite all of the puking, she has to take in protein and carbohydrate-based foods. But while sticking to this, if you wish to have a meat-based protein in your diet, make certain that the meat is not undercooked. Even fish that's high in mercury content is an absolute no.

Week 10

This is a big week in terms of medical terminology. What has been referred to as an embryo all this while can now finally be called a fetus. While medically it just refers to the distinction between gestational age, for you and I, it might make more sense to look at it slightly differently. While the embryo is still forming all the basic human organs, a fetus is like a miniature version of a human baby. This is to say that all the organs that the baby will need once it comes out, are already formed when it becomes a fetus. Though the organs are quite basic, the fetus' vulnerability will keep decreasing as time progresses.

Your Baby's Growth

The fetus starts showing signs of the baby's sex. If it's a boy, the testes are starting to appear and the baby is already starting to produce testosterone. The baby also has started showing signs of teeth formation below the gum line. But remember, these teeth won't break out until the baby is about six months of age. As bones and cartilage in the skeletal structure develop more and more, the baby's elbows and knees start functioning. Can you believe that the baby's arms are already flexing by now?! How awesome is that?

Your Partner's Experience

The fun pregnancy symptoms that your partner has been experiencing all along are here to stay. But as if she wasn't having enough fun, her body may decide to drop another pregnancy bomb, or rather hold off dropping anything at all! Constipation is a symptom your partner will frequently experience as her bowels refuse to function smoothly. A few things that may help are eating enough fiber, drinking lots of water, and getting on her feet for some physical activity.

This is also the time when your partner's baby bump may start showing. This is not quite noticeable until you consciously decide to look at it. Also, baby bumps come in all shapes and sizes. So, just because your partner isn't "showing" as much as someone else isn't something to worry about for now. Your partner may also experience what is known as round ligament pain. These are nothing but the growing pains of an expanding belly.

Another physical change that may come on is the appearance of bluish veins all over your partner's abdomen and breasts. These veins, again, are nothing to worry about and are just a sign that your partner's body is expanding its blood circulation network to accommodate the circulatory needs of the baby as well.

What You Can Do

The first thing you need to do is be there with her for all the antenatal tests. Testing can be a time filled with anxiety and apprehension. Make sure she doesn't have to battle out those overwhelming emotions all by herself.

Also, if you haven't already, this might be a good time to start documenting the pregnancy as the external signs also become more apparent. This means that now it's also time to start shopping for some maternity clothing. This first outward sign that her body is going to be changing tremendously, can make it all too real for your partner, triggering anxiety. Find romantic ways to let her know that she is beautiful as ever by maybe leaving her random post-it reminders here and there.

The lifestyle choices that you have already made, for instance, healthy eating, ample sleep, and appropriate levels of workout, will continue and may need tweaking as per your partner's needs. Taking a yoga class might be a bonus that brings physical activity as well as emotional tranquility for your partner.

Week 11

By this week the baby is about one and a half inches long. The head is still disproportionately large as compared to the rest of the body making up for almost half the body size. Now is also the time to start discussing the big reveal to your friends and family as you are reaching the third month's end.

Your Baby's Growth

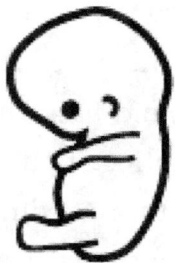

During this week, your baby is developing hair follicles not just on the head but all over the body. These hair follicles will eventually result in hairy growth when the baby is born to ensure some protection against extreme temperature fluctuations.

Fingernails and toenails are forming this week. In the later part of the pregnancy, the baby will start growing nails even while in the womb. If it's a girl, ovaries start developing now. The baby now has a tongue and a palate in the mouth, and nipples start becoming apparent.

An exciting thing for parents is to learn that their baby is now doing all sorts of gymnastics within the mother's body, be it rolling forward, stretching, and even somersaults. But again, these are likely too weak for your partner to feel at this moment.

Your Partner's Experience

The great news is that by now morning sickness has faded out for most women. But hold onto your excitement because the morning sickness is likely to be only replaced by bloating and gas. This is normal because the body is now adapting its digestive mechanism to slow the process so that maximum nutrients can be absorbed for the mother as well as the baby. As beneficial as this is to the fast-growing baby, it can be quite unpleasant for your partner.

Add this to the growing baby bump and your partner will likely find getting into her old jeans pretty uncomfortable thereby worsening the unpleasant experience. This phase might be a little tricky because your partner is lurking in the still-too-early-to-be-in-maternity-clothes period.

What You Can Do

By this week, she will be getting up in the middle of the night far too often for you to not notice. While it is completely understandable that you cannot stay up all night with her all the time, one thing that can help is installing some nightlights in the bathroom and on her way there. Before going off to sleep make sure you clear out the path for her so that she doesn't trip while on any of her bathroom trips.

As you'll realize, your partner is probably pretty miserable at this point with the physical and emotional symptoms. Recording the baby bump with a pregnancy photo shoot might be a welcome distraction from all that's going on. Also, planning a pregnancy reveal to your friends and family can be a fun activity both of you can undertake.

Week 12

You are almost at the end of the first trimester. As the external signs of pregnancy become more and more real, as a new father you might find yourself coming into your role quite naturally. I know that I did for sure whenever my wife was pregnant. I mean, sure, I feel that way about my kids and wife all the time but something about your partner's growing baby bump just makes you feel protective of her and the baby.

Your Baby's Growth

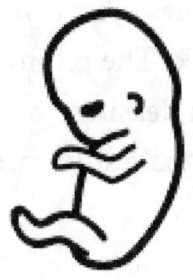

By this time your baby is about a couple of inches long, almost the size of a lime. The baby is crossing some major milestones here. By the end of this week, the fetus has all of the major organs in place. Though it's nowhere close to the physical maturity that they need to reach yet, all the systems are in place.

Also, by now, the baby's intestines which were crowding the umbilical space have now retracted into the baby's abdomen. The baby's bone marrow has also started developing white blood cells which are crucial in protecting against infection. The baby can now respond to external stimuli. Certain reflexes like sucking also set in during this week and the baby is likely to move spontaneously. But of course, the fetus is too small for the mother to feel anything yet.

If you have been excited about having a kid, think about having a grandkid someday, someday being the keyword! I know what you are thinking—your plate is a little too full to be thinking of 30 years in the future. Well, guess what your unborn baby's brain is already working on this week; The pituitary gland in the fetus' brain is already releasing hormones that might someday allow your baby to reproduce and become a parent.

Your Partner's Experience

As the end of the first trimester draws closer, your partner may experience just a tad bit of relief in terms of her physical and emotional symptoms, though this may vary widely across individuals. While every now and then she may experience indigestion and find herself passing gas, the discomfort is likely to be lesser as compared to the last few weeks.

But just like some symptoms are fading out, some new ones may arrive to keep her company. One of these would be dizziness. As progesterone continues to be secreted, it attempts to increase the blood supply to the baby sometimes at the cost of a slower blood supply to your partner. This low blood pressure can induce light-headedness especially when she makes sudden movements.

What You Can Do

It's likely that in the midst of all this, your partner may not exactly be up for sex. But a diminished libido can be an actual consequence of the good old hormones. Of course, the other possibility is that the sex drive may see a steep spike in some women. But whichever category your partner falls into, thinking of creative romantic ways to reconnect may earn you some quality brownie points. If you have kept track of her cravings, for instance, surprising her with her favorite bite-sized treats in bed can be a great idea.

If it's the flu season, that is October to May, you should encourage your partner to get that flu shot. If you're worried about the side effects, you can breathe easily because research supports its safety for pregnant mothers'.

You'll also do well to keep a tip or two in mind to help her through her dizzy spells. During these, encourage her to keep her head in between her knees and take deep breaths. If she is wearing slightly tight jeans, she can unbutton them for a while. Get her something to drink and eat if she is up for it. Sometimes, a sweet can also help in raising blood glucose levels instantly.

One of these days, you can take her out shopping for loose, flowy dresses and tops and whatever she may like. Believe me, the fashion industry out there is much more evolved than we men think it to be. Get her clothes that make her feel beautiful and confident enough to rock that baby bump.

Week 13

The week you have been waiting for is finally here. The first trimester is drawing to a close and will be over within a few days. The highlight is, of course, the drastic drop in the risk of miscarriage. Along with this though, the baby bump is becoming harder to conceal even with the loose-fitting clothes. Get ready for big things ahead!

Your Baby's Growth

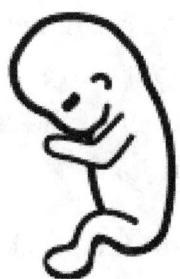

The baby is now almost the size of a lemon. The body proportions continue to change as the head is now one-third of the baby's entire length. The fetus even has fingerprints by now. The baby is also witnessing the development of vocal cords this week. The baby will soon find these very handy in keeping you up at night with crying and screaming bloody murder! I am kidding; these chords will also be responsible for the babbling sounds that the baby makes when you are playing with it.

Now that the basic systems are in place, major variations are seen across fetuses in the rate of their growth and development. The placenta has continued to grow and soon will take over the entire function of nourishing the fetus.

Your Partner's Experience

Your partner's mood swings are going to be hard on you but remember they are much harder on her. Imagine feeling like you are in heaven one moment and hell the next! Talk about extremes! And since you are the partner and the father of the child you will likely be on the receiving end of it all.

Constipation will continue to contribute to this irritability too. Vaginal discharge which we discussed in the earlier weeks will continue and may even increase. As long as the discharge is colorless or milky and odorless, you both are in the clear. If not, it's best to consult your healthcare provider.

With the fetus getting bigger, your partner's breasts are starting to prepare for breastfeeding when the baby arrives. During this week, they start producing colostrum which is the first stage of breast milk.

A symptom that may arise often is headaches. This might seem like we are exaggerating the symptoms a little, it's just a headache after all! But try getting through the headache without any meds and remedies and you'll realize how debilitating these "simple" headaches can be. With any non-prescribed medicines and substances out of bounds, your partner will have to battle these out all on her own.

One good thing you'll notice is your partner's fatigue is decreasing and she is coming back to her original energy levels. But even if that's the case, remember that strenuous physical activity, especially lifting things is still a no-go.

What You Can Do

Help your partner plan meals and portion sizes. You can make weekly plans for several small meals a day rather than having three big ones. This is likely to give her at least some relief through her indigestion and constipation. Another tip is to ingest as much fiber as possible and sometimes that may include eating unpeeled fruits. Making sure she is stocked up on fluids and fiber and that she is eating on time is your best shot at relieving some of the physical symptoms. Apart from that, making sure she has some time to herself where she can relax should be on your to-do list.

THE DATING SCAN

Start getting used to a new meaning that dating will bring in your life because it sure is not the dating you have engaged in with your partner thus far. The dating scan is the ultrasound test that can help determine how far along you are in your pregnancy. Remember you enquired with your doctor about testing somewhere in the seventh week? It's likely your doctor suggested weeks 10-14 for when this testing can start.

The dating scan might be a part of a larger subset of tests that aim at identifying chromosomal defects. This scan itself takes about 20 minutes and may just require your partner to have a full bladder.

There are various kinds of tests at this point including non-invasive prenatal testing (NIPT) which is merely a blood test and chorionic villus sampling (CVS). While NIPT is highly accurate in detecting down syndrome cases (almost 99%), CVS is slightly more advanced and can detect additional defects like spina bifida, muscular dystrophy, hemophilia, etc. These tests take a couple of weeks to give you the results.

THE TRAUMA OF MISCARRIAGES

Though we talk about the drastically decreased risk of pregnancy, I feel it is just as essential to have a conversation about miscarriages. Of course, this is not to induce any sort of negativity but the topic of miscarriages is so hushed up that couples often never get the chance to process them fully. I know how difficult it was for me and my wife when this unfortunate event shook our worlds. Though I cannot undo the pain of this loss for myself or any of you, it is important to talk about it.

When this happened to us, we were way past the first trimester, almost in week 26. We never really understood what caused it but my wife went into early labor and the baby did not make it. One thing I know as a parent is that I didn't love that unborn child any less at week 12 than I did at week 26. Parenthood hardly cares about how old the child is.

The point is, we felt terribly shattered and that loss will never be forgotten. Since by then everyone knew of the pregnancy, we were showered with love and support each step of the way by friends and family alike. What surprised us, though, was that friends reached out with their own stories of loss and pain. It was only then that we realized how common miscarriages are. And what was more was that these couples hardly had anyone to talk to when they were going through it.

Of course, this is a call that you and your partner will take together, but I urge you to think about who you'd like to know about your pregnancy even before the first trimester is up. God forbid, if something goes wrong, you'll need someone to lean on. Maybe tell your parents or closest friends, people who you can truly rely on in case of a physical as well as emotional emergency.

Another thing you need to be clear about is it's not your fault. I remember both of us thinking constantly if it was something that we did that led to this. The truth is as much as you try to follow the prescribed to-do list, there will still be things that are out of your control and understanding. That sucks, I know, but all you can do is allow yourself to feel the pain and keep moving forward. That does not mean you forget the loss, chances you never will, but trying to rebuild your life with the shattered pieces is your only choice.

5

THE FOURTH MONTH

The second trimester is here and your partner is likely to have an easier time coping with the pregnancy. As the physical and emotional symptoms get easier for your partner, she will have more energy to think about fun stuff like shopping for the baby, or planning and readying the nursery.

A highlight of this trimester is the gender reveal. This is, of course, only if you care to find out. Many parents may choose not to and wait for the joyful surprise at the time of delivery. But if you do give in to the temptation, you can even plan for a gender reveal for your friends and family.

THE WEEK-BY-WEEK PROGRESS

This is also the time that you would be preparing for the actual birth. This is to say, you and your partner will discuss more specific details of the birthing plan and figure out the best logistics possible. You can look through the various options mentioned before to figure out the one that suits your needs the best.

Week 14

By now, you are likely to have announced this to your friends and family. If you are a first-time parent you are likely to be flooded with advice from all sides. Remember that just as individuals, no two parents are alike. So, while there's merit to some of this advice and criticism, not all of it will apply to you personally. Be careful about what advice you pick and choose.

Your Baby's Growth

During this week, the baby is almost as big as a baseball. The hair follicles that developed earlier are now sprouting up with fine hair called lanugo. The hand and leg coordination is getting much better. While the baby has been exhibiting some jerky movements for some time, now the baby seems to be on the go all the time. The movements are also quite fluid and smooth. New positions are also on the cards as the baby learns to stretch a little rather than curl up in a ball at all times.

The proportions get better as the baby's body length increases more compared to the head. Till now the baby looked like a big round ball joined directly to the tiny body. But now, the neck that will support the baby's head has started developing. The kidneys have also assumed their functional positions.

Your Partner's Experience

Your partner would have to brace for a lot more poking and prodding in the coming months. The second trimester brings a lot more doctor appointments as the healthcare provider keeps an eye on blood pressure, weight gain, fetal development, etc.

Round ligament pain is persistent as the uterus cramps out her abdomen. Heartburn and flatulence are two particularly uncomfortable symptoms that will be on the rise during this week and probably for the rest of the pregnancy. As funny as it may seem to you, make sure your partner feels the same way about your fart-jokes before laughing it off in front of others or even just between yourselves.

Emotionally, the process of "nesting" might well be on its way as your partner strips the house down shelf by shelf and finds ways to reorganize everything to prepare for the baby's arrival.

What You Can Do

Though you might find it difficult to keep up with the tasks your partner is accomplishing currently, you can certainly spearhead some tasks like setting up the nursery on your own. But make sure both your ideas are incorporated because this is gonna be "baby central" for some time now.

This is a good time to inquire about the paternity leave policies at your workplace. This includes leaves not only after the baby comes but also when you accompany your partner for the prenatal appointments. If at all these aren't an option in your company you might want to plan ahead and save up on your leaves; that can come in handy during the pregnancy.

Week 15

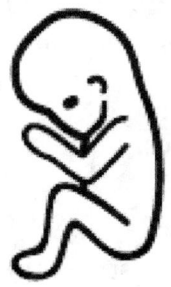

The highlight of this week would have to be the possibility that your partner can feel the baby's movements. However, with so much going on in her abdomen region like constipation, gas, and round ligament pain, this fractional sensation may just go unnoticed. Another exciting development is finding the gender of the baby that we spoke of at the beginning of the chapter.

Your Baby's Growth

You can now breathe a little easier because the baby is surely breathing on its own. The lungs are stronger than before but still quite primitive. Nonetheless, they can take over the breathing function effectively.

The baby is now almost as big as a pear but is yet to develop the adult opaque skin giving you a see-through view of the developing blood vessels among other things. The bones are becoming more and more opaque with the process of their formation underway, called ossification.

If you were to observe the baby at this stage, you might just mistake it for a gymnastic instructor with the constant movement in the womb. But in actuality, this is just practice for the world outside the safety of the womb.

The taste buds, which in the coming years, are going to make it very difficult for you to feed your baby healthy broccoli, are developing during this week. All in all a pretty busy week!

Your Partner's Experience

If you thought pregnancy brain was just a humorous play on a pregnant woman's state of mind, you are in for a surprise. Pregnancy brain is quite real. Your partner is going to be losing stuff every few moments and this in itself can be quite frustrating.

In addition to the digestive discomfort, the hormones are causing some problems in her mouth for now. Bleeding gums and dental conditions are also quite common in women during pregnancy.

Braxton Hicks when experienced for the first time can be quite overwhelming. I remember the first time this happened to my wife; we were scared out of our minds. Though we knew about these contractions, we still couldn't keep from making a panicked call to the doctor. These are likely to come around this week especially if it's your partner's first pregnancy. These false alarms are her body's way of preparing for the D-day. In the beginning, these are quite likely to be painless but may increase in intensity as weeks progress.

What You Can Do

The baby anxiety might kick in at this point. Especially when your partner is all over the place due to the pregnancy brain, she can have major self-doubt about caring for the baby. At this point, again, talking about her fears and reassuring her of the fact that you are going to be with her every step of the way can be quite comforting.

If you are the gender reveal party kind then you should probably get started on it with your partner. This can be a welcome distraction for her from all the self-doubt and maybe a fun activity for both of you.

Checking with the doctor to see if her weight is in a healthy range is another thing you need to check in on during your appointments.

Week 16

As the pregnancy becomes more and more obvious, your partner will find that more people approach her with advice, instructions and even belly rubs that she never asked for. It is around this time that you and your partner will have to talk about the boundary setting regarding what is ok and what makes her uncomfortable, regarding people touching her or offering advice.

Your Baby's Growth

The baby is now about five inches long, that's almost the size of an avocado. An intriguing highlight is that though its eyes are closed, the fetus can respond to external light and move its eyes from side to side.

Though ears have been in place for a while, it's during this time that the bones in the ear are forming and the baby will soon be able to perceive and respond to sound. The baby is now also able to hold its head a little straighter. Though it doesn't have hair yet, the scalp is already forming patterns that vary from individual to individual.

Your Partner's Experience

The uterus is now the size of a papaya. Ever tried hiding papaya under your shirt? It's quite the task. By now, hiding the pregnancy may just not be possible. Baby movements are quite frequent. You'd think the magic of that feeling would fade out after the first few kicks, but you'll be surprised!

Your partner will likely put on quite a few pounds around this time. If she ensures that she is eating right, then she can be sure that the pounds will likely shed off in the long run. Yet gaining weight can be intimidating for some women.

The good thing though is that she has a much better handle on her emotions. Her mood swings have stabilized a great deal and it is less likely that you will find her crying in the bathroom because you kept her snack jar in a different place! Better moods mean better coping with her own body changes as well.

Apart from the regular Braxton Hicks contractions, bleeding gums, tender, and growing breasts, etc. a stuffy nose might be added to the mix of symptoms that your partner is experiencing.

What You Can Do

Tell her she is beautiful every day because she is even with that extra weight and the baby bump, especially with those things. That is the first thing you need to do. Also, make sure she is getting her nutrition from healthy calories rather than empty ones.

As the size of her uterus increases, her back is going to be overworked all the time. Getting her a prenatal massage may help relieve the tension in her muscles. Also, encouraging her for gentle Yoga classes or mild pilates sessions may help with the back pain too.

If you haven't had your genetic testing done, this might be a good time to prepare for what's known as a quad scan.

Another fun thing you want to do is set up a baby registry through which your loved ones can give you things that you might actually find helpful when the baby arrives. You'll want to add to that list basic items like a stroller, a car seat, crib, blankets, baby monitor, diapers, baby clothing like onesies, bibs, leg warmers, etc. You can look at the checklist I gave you at the beginning of this book for ideas.

Week 17

Though your baby is already a looker with all its features in place now, it is still pretty skinny and not yet cute in the conventional sense of the word. This week the baby's fat proportions are growing. Now, the baby can also respond to external auditory stimuli.

Your Baby's Growth

The bones continue to ossify and replace cartilage. As the baby is growing, so are its nourishment needs. This can be seen by the continued strengthening of the umbilical cord which carries the main nutrition supply to the baby from the mother.

The baby is also developing sweat glands by now and is still keeping busy with the reflex practice like sucking, swallowing, etc. Though, technically, there is nothing to feed on in the traditional sense yet, practicing these reflexes will help the baby ingest the breastmilk or formula once the umbilical cord is cut at birth.

Your Partner's Experience

The nasal congestion may worsen as her sensitivity to allergens increases. You might hear her snoring too in bed. Another symptom that is experienced by many women is a bloody nose. This is nothing to worry about most of the time and is usually just a sign that her body is circulating more blood than before. The same vaginal discharge we spoke of earlier is on the rise and is normal.

The growing belly is also making it more difficult for her to get around as she becomes more clumsy. Your partner may also have stretch marks as souvenirs of the pregnancy. These may be hereditary and many women find these quite upsetting. Ensuring that the weight gain is gradual rather than in bursts, might help in keeping the stretch marks to a minimum. As for me and my wife, we consider it a badge of honor and bravery, and she wears them proudly.

Backaches get intense to the point of developing sciatica which is a sharp shooting pain in the back. Your partner may also experience gestational arthritis leading to numbing joint pains. The dental troubles are nowhere near over for your partner as her teeth loosen owing to the crazy hormone tricks. Now might be a good time to visit that dentist that you have been avoiding for a while.

What You Can Do

As her skin stretches some weird skin conditions may pop in ranging from dryness to rashes. She may even develop some temporary moles. Buy her some coconut oil and sunscreen to avoid these.

Ensure that she eats a lot of calcium-rich food because the baby is drawing on her calcium reserves for the ossification of bones.

The previously discussed pregnancy brain is having a raging party in your partner's head. Be patient with her as she loses everything she can possibly lose—phone, charger, keys, purse. You name it and by now she is quite likely to have forgotten that item at least once. This can be frustrating especially when you have to leave the house for an appointment. You can minimize delays by factoring in these delays and getting ready to leave a little earlier than is actually required.

And just like that your fourth month is over! This may be a good time to start registering yourself and your partner for childbirth classes.

6

THE FIFTH MONTH

The ticker is ticking and it's four down, five to go. As the baby is now responding to sound with movements of all kinds, the pregnancy might just feel more real. Especially for your partner the reminder that she is carrying a living, breathing human within her can be almost intimidating.

THE WEEK-BY-WEEK PROGRESS

It is often seen that the baby can time her movements perfectly when the mother is resting, making it harder for the mother to clock in some much-needed rest. But as this month will draw to a close the baby's erratic sleep and wake schedules settle into a more predictable pattern.

Week 18

The ultrasounds this month become even more exciting as they start catching the baby's actions like yawning and hiccuping. The gender reveal that you planned for, if at all you planned for anything fancy, could happen around this time. While a decade back no one really thought of gender reveals as an event, today many parents come up with quite creative ideas of letting everyone on this joy. If you are falling short of ideas you can always get some inspiration from social media.

Your Baby's Growth

Though you have already found the gender of the baby based on the beginnings of genitalia sometime back, this is the time when your baby develops the genitals in a much more noticeable manner. If it's a girl, the reproductive system is beginning to form with the formation of fallopian tubes.

Around this time, the baby's nervous system is also developing rapidly. The nerves that began forming at such a fast pace in the initial weeks are now getting myelinated. That is to say, the nerves are being covered with sheaths of a special substance called myelin which make it possible for neural signals to be transmitted at a brilliant speed.

With the ears in their complete final shape, the baby's listening capacities are also greatly increased. While it could already react to external sound stimuli, now it is also becoming more adept at picking up internal sounds like the mother's hiccups or the faint growling of her stomach.

Your Partner's Experience

While dizziness, flatulence, and acid reflux continue to cause her discomfort, your partner is likely to be in much better spirits now. Her fatigue is gone and she might seem to have a new bout of energy coursing through her. She may have occasional panic moments about the coming baby but these are likely to be more because of the approaching due date rather than hormonal fluctuations.

A new symptom that your partner might get introduced to, is edema which is swollen feet and ankles and also intense spasms often known as charley horse. Stretch marks are also increasing at a steady pace.

What You Can Do

As her nutrition needs increase, you might have to wear the chef's hat even more than usual, to make sure that she is eating healthy. But you both mustn't take the healthy lifestyle to extremes with a heavy workout. In fact, you might have to urge your partner to stop some workout routines that require her to lie down on her back altogether.

Give her a foot rub before she heads to bed. Also, try to encourage her to stretch her feet, that might just decrease the intensity of those calf spasms that she has been experiencing in the middle of the night.

Week 19

This week the baby might get into a growth spurt phase and grow suddenly overnight. These growth spurts will be seen even as the baby arrives and steps into early childhood.

Your Baby's Growth

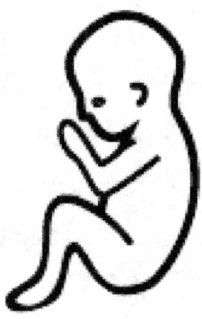

Your baby is now almost six inches long. As time passes by, the baby is now getting comfy in the mother's womb. Apart from developing the reflexes more and more, now the baby develops a greasy layer on its skin known as vernix caseosa. To understand its function, think of your fingers after you wash the dishes or when you take an extra-long bath. The fingers most likely get wrinkled as they are immersed in water. Imagine dipping them in there for nine months straight. The same would happen to the baby if not for this oily layer that repels fluid and keeps the baby's skin as soft as possible. It also protects the baby from infections while in the womb.

The baby is now the size of a big mango and has a much more proportionate body with legs that are longer than the arms and head that is more proportionate than before.

Your Partner's Experience

The mother may experience a sharp increase in her appetite aligned with the baby's growth spurts. We may not have much to add to the symptom list this week but the older symptoms might be going at full force—backache, spasm, round ligament pain, nasal congestion, stretch marks, dizzy spells, and so on.

What You Can Do

Studies have proven that fathers tend to have lower levels of testosterone and estradiol during pregnancy. That means you are as tuned in to this pregnancy as your partner. So, every once in a while remember to take care of yourself as well. As far as your partner goes, make sure your pantry is stocked up so that whenever she has her hunger pangs, you can put together a quick sandwich, hearty and healthy. Also, keep following up on the plenty of fluids and fiber rules. A great way to show your solidarity is by giving up on junk food yourself as well.

Make sure she has a comfortable pair of shoes. Heels and wedges need to exit for a while. With her sense of balance a little off due to the growing belly and her backache, flats are going to be her most comfortable option.

Week 20

If you are watching the weeks like a hawk, you will realize that this week you have crossed the halfway mark. Go ahead, give your partner a celebratory treat (it has to be something that she likes) and you have definitely earned a pat on your back too for all the heavy-lifting you have been doing around the house.

Your Baby's Growth

The baby is now almost the length of a banana, almost ten inches long. Gender development continues this week too. If it's a girl her uterus is developing right now and she already has a lifetime worth of eggs stowed away in her ovaries. While for now, it's somewhere around seven million primitive eggs which will eventually reduce to one or two million before birth. If it's a boy, the testicles that made an appearance earlier and have been growing since make their journey from the abdomen downwards. The scrotum is still developing.

Your Partner's Experience

While her heartburn and flatulence are continuing symptoms, her sex drive might be in top gear around now. The belly is not just growing but is becoming rounder too. As the abdomen stretches to accommodate the growing uterus, the appearance of her navel may also change whereby her inward belly button suddenly starts protruding outward. This isn't anything to worry about and the navel will go to its original look when she delivers.

What You Can Do

This week has what is known as the 20-week anatomy scan to monitor the baby's growth till this point. Make sure these appointments are strictly adhered to.

As the delivery date comes closer, you'd want to also start thinking of names for the baby. If you already know the gender, this is even easier, just pick the top five names that you like. Even if you don't have the gender, you can still pick the top five for each gender and finalize on the top names that you both agree on. Remember that both of you can veto a name that you don't like. And the vetoes can go on for quite some time.

Week 21

By now the baby's movements are almost graceful and have replaced the jerky, uncoordinated movements. The kicks and punches are strong and frequent.

Your Baby's Growth

The baby is almost as long as a carrot now, inching closer to a foot. It weighs a solid one pound at this stage. While the placenta is still the major source of nutrition, the baby is also hooked on to the taste of amniotic fluid. This means that whatever the mother is having at this point, is likely to be the baby's favorite flavor.

The baby's looks are now changing with the eyebrows appearing on its face. If it's a girl, she is also developing a vagina and the vaginal canal at this point. Till now your baby's liver and spleen have been working over-time to make blood cells but now the bone marrow is developed enough to chip in too.

Your Partner's Experience

With the amount of activity that she is feeling in her womb, your partner may find it hard to believe that the baby is sleeping at all. But the truth is the fetus is sleeping quite a lot, almost as much as a newborn.

As the baby's taste buds develop more and more, your partner would need to be more mindful about the food she ingests. As the taste of the amniotic fluid changes daily based on the diet, the baby will also be quick to pick up on the different flavors. Even research suggests that the baby is likely to eat more of the food that resembles what it has tasted in the uterus.

Your partner might also experience a condition called preeclampsia that is specific to the duration of pregnancy. The mother may experience high blood pressure and even exhibit signs of strain on organs like the liver and kidneys. It is best to consult your doctor about this but in most cases, this condition alleviates after the pregnancy is through.

Varicose veins and spider veins are other conditions that might make an entry.

What You Can Do

Tiny gestures like helping your partner elevate her feet when watching TV, for instance, might reduce the pain a great deal. Also, remind her every now and then to sleep on her left side as this facilitates smoother circulation.

If you have been feeling like you always miss your baby's best moves, then it's time to get your partner to kick back and relax because the baby is most likely to be on the go when mommy is resting. Also, the best time to feel those kicks is when your partner pops something healthy in her mouth as the rise in blood glucose level increases the likelihood of the baby's movement.

Week 22

If you don't already, now is the time you need to watch the mother's environment as minutely as possible because from within her womb, your baby is making much more sense of the world than before. By now, the baby is pretty much the skinny version of the baby that's going to come out. The baby is now getting closer to the time when it might even survive a premature birth and is likely to get there in a couple of weeks.

Your Baby's Growth

The baby is getting bigger and is now almost the size of a papaya. By this week, the baby has started experimenting with its strengthened sense of touch. It's holding and even tugging on the umbilical cord. This is significant not only because the baby is developing motor reflexes but also because of the underlying brain development that is leading to these motor changes.

Even though the baby's eyes are sealed shut, it can still perceive light and dark. You can test this for yourself by shining a flashlight on your partner's womb and there will likely be immediate movement in response to that light. The baby is now also responding more strongly to the sounds it hears and it feels stressed when exposed to loud noises despite these noises being muffled.

Your Partner's Experience

By this time your partner might be feeling like Bigfoot as her feet have gained in half or even full shoe size. In addition to its role in relaxing the blood vessels for increased blood supply that we saw earlier, relaxin also helps in loosening the bones, muscles, and ligaments, specifically pelvic bones. But unfortunately, it cannot distinguish between pelvic and other ligaments. The part that will be the most affected by this is your partner's feet. And often it might not go back to the original size even after the pregnancy is over.

As her belly gets bigger, she might find it increasingly difficult to find a comfortable sleeping position, thereby causing some irritability. Her skin may start showing pigmentation and a dark line may appear on her belly.

What You Can Do

Buy her a pregnancy pillow that can act as a sleeping aid to help her sleep through the night. Start a conversation about breastfeeding and see what her opinions on it are. If she is planning to breastfeed, some shopping might be in order. Remind her about nursing bras and shirts that make it a little more convenient to breastfeed in public. A breast pump might be a worthy investment too.

7

THE SIXTH MONTH

Whoa! You have made it to six out of the nine months and are going strong. That's your second trimester which counts for two-thirds of the pregnancy. Though the finish line is getting closer, remember that it's also getting harder for your partner to get around with that ever-increasing belly. That means she has to up her resting period and you need to up your housekeeping skills.

THE WEEK-BY-WEEK PROGRESS

Though it may seem like this is just the month of waiting around, the baby is still crossing some major milestones off the list. Also, since your partner is probably in a good mood most of the time, this might be the best time to plan ahead. Living with a baby isn't the same as living without one. That seems like a pretty obvious thing to say but I remember for me, the significance didn't sink in until we started thinking of baby-proofing the apartment. It was only after we started talking about it that we realized that the tiniest things we never even thought of, mattered a great deal. Though the baby-proofing won't come in until later, this might be the time to ponder over all the facets of your life that may need to be realigned with the baby's arrival.

Week 23

Brace yourself for a solid growth spurt over the coming month. Up until now, even with all the development, the baby was growing through, it still had ample space in the uterus. But as the baby's size grows and the mother's uterus is stretched to its limit, things might start getting a little crammed in.

Your Baby's Growth

The skin that may have seemed a little wrinkled and saggy before is now becoming taut and soft because of the formation of a fatty layer underneath. This will significantly impact both size and weight. The blood vessels, specifically the arteries and veins are also developing under the skin resulting in a pinkish-red hue (for all skin colors). In addition to this, the blood vessels are also developing in the lungs to prepare for respiration when the baby gets out. By now the placenta has also been fully formed and has completely taken over the function of nourishment of the baby.

Your Partner's Experience

As the uterus dominates the bladder, the chances of a urinary tract infection increase. Though there are things that can be done to reduce the risk, your partner is likely to be constantly aware of it.

With all the oncoming symptoms impacting her feet, back, teeth, nose, she may not even realize what's happening in her hands. With the increasing swelling pressure, she might experience a tingling sensation in her wrists. This is especially if she works with computers all day. She might also find herself wanting to gorge on every edible thing in the kitchen as she is eating for two now.

What You Can Do

Now would be a good time for your partner to talk to the HR department in her office and plan for the maternity leave. This in itself can cause some anxiety about losing touch with her work or even about the fact that she might not stay at the top of her boss' minds. If she experiences such anxiety, try to give a calm, patient listening ear without jumping on to the legality and technicality of it all. Of course, it could be important to remind her of that as well but understand the underlying baby vs. career struggle she might be going through.

Make sure she is having ample fluids and water to steer clear of the UTI danger. The water levels will also keep her blood volume and the amniotic fluid content at optimum levels. Also, don't forget to stock up on healthy snacks like veggies, nuts, fruits, etc. when your partner turns into a hungry panda.

Week 24

This week will see some new symptoms for the mother, but she and you will hardly care. This is because this week brings with it the wonderful news of the fetus viability. This means that the baby has all systems in place like a normal baby would and can thus survive even if the mother goes into early labor. Almost half to three-fourths of the babies born at this stage make it. Though I have learned from our experience that preterm delivery is still unpredictably stressful, crossing this milestone is nonetheless a huge relief.

Your Baby's Growth

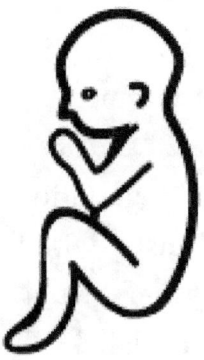

Now that the baby is physically equipped to perform all the functions, the next few months will be dedicated to the fortification of those organ systems. The baby's hearing is now strong enough to perceive sounds that it will even recognize after birth. The fat deposition isn't over as yet and will continue for some time to come.

Your Partner's Experience

Mom continues to have a party within her body with swollen feet, backache, nasal congestion, acid reflux, all grooving to the music of her flatulence. The tingling wrists from the last week have now graduated into full-blown carpal tunnel syndrome which is the new guest to the rager your partner is hosting. Her uterus is now almost as big and round as a soccer ball which might mean that she has to put in the extra effort while getting up and sitting down.

What You Can Do

Your doctor might recommend going for a glucose test somewhere between 24 to 28 weeks of pregnancy to keep an eye out for gestational diabetes that we mentioned earlier. Consult with your doctor about the necessary changes in her diet that might bring those sugar levels back to normal.

As the D-day draws closer, it's best to keep all the things you will need when you go to the hospital, packed and ready. If your partner does go into labor at an unexpected time, these will prove to be a lifesaver. This can have your basic stuff to help you and your partner get through the hospital stay—a few comfy clothes, chargers, some downloaded entertainment, feminine pads, and so on.

Week 25

This week is more of what's already present. Though new developments might be few, the ongoing maturation is crucial for the preparation for the baby's first day out.

Your Baby's Growth

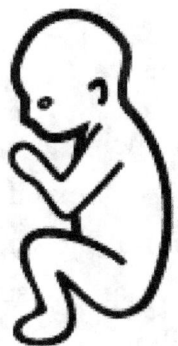

The baby's appearance will significantly improve as time goes and the layer of fat increases, thus getting rid of the wrinkly and translucent skin that has been present for a long time.

The baby's size is comparable to acorn squash, about 13 inches long. This week the capillary, or blood vessel, development is on a roll. Along with those under the skin, the ones in the air sacs are also developing leading to the fortification we spoke of. The baby would still not be able to breathe on its own but it's surely getting there.

The baby is also developing a startle reflex which will later be referred to as the Moro reflex. Once the baby is born the loud noises it hears make it spread its arms, then pulls back in, and start crying. This reflex helps the baby to stay close to the mother thereby increasing the chances of its survival.

Your Partner's Experience

The Mommy is experiencing all of the already existing symptoms. Her varicose veins, if she has them, might get worse and make a full-blown entrance in the form of hemorrhoids. This can cause pain and can even result in rectal bleeding. These are not particularly dangerous and can be managed with certain pelvic floor exercises as well as a fibrous diet.

As if all her symptoms weren't enough, she now may have symphysis pubis dysfunction. No, don't worry, it's not as scary as it sounds. This is the pelvic pain that your partner might be feeling as the pelvic joints become unaligned due to pelvic relaxation.

She might also be experiencing restless leg syndrome where you have a strong desire to move it. This may be significant because it might relate to iron deficiency.

What You Can Do

Keep a food journal and encourage her to keep making notes in it. Whenever you are around, you can make notes for her. This will give you a reference point when consulting your doctor. Encourage your partner to keep the exercise schedule going to help her through the aches.

Now may be a good time to start discussing her doula needs. A doula and a midwife are not the same. A doula is there to support your partner through the emotional journey but has no medical training. Research suggests that mothers who have doulas are more likely to have smoother deliveries. It's certainly something worth considering.

While you are at it also finalize all the details of the birth such as whether it would be medicated or unmedicated. Also think about where it would happen, which hospital or birth center or just at home. The financial feasibility of all this would also have to be considered.

Week 26

If it's a boy then this is the week that the boy makes an entry into manhood—well, at least as much as he can while crammed up in his mother's womb. By now the baby weighs almost two pounds.

Your Baby's Growth

All this while the baby's eyes have been completely sealed. All the eye movements have been from behind the eyelids. Now, however, they are starting to open up and eyelashes are starting to form. The irises are still not pigmented. The baby's nails are also growing and the baby will likely have sharp nails by the time it comes out.

Along with this, the baby's lungs are also growing stronger and the chances of its survival increase tremendously with each passing day. The senses which have already made the appearance keep getting better with time.

Your Partner's Experience

Braxton-Hicks contractions continue as her body prepares to give birth. The belly, of course, keeps increasing making your partner uncomfortable and sometimes even irritable. Her heartburn continues to grow worse too.

Out of nowhere, your partner might suddenly start having difficulty with her vision. She may experience blurred vision, and dry eyes as the pregnancy hormones decrease tear production. Headaches and migraines continue to ruin her peace of mind. But despite the physical discomfort, your partner is still likely to be in an upbeat mood.

What You Can Do

As the due date approaches, the Braxton Hicks contractions can get more emotionally stressful because it may feel like she is going into preterm labor. Make sure you talk to her about her anxieties and ask her if there is anything that you can do to alleviate her physical or emotional discomfort.

Also, be sure to consult your healthcare provider for complaints regarding vision because there is a small chance that those might be related to preeclampsia or the heightened blood pressure condition that we discussed earlier.

Week 27

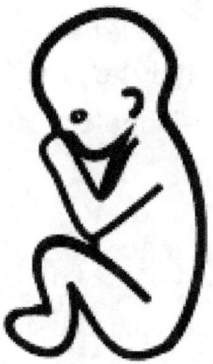

This week you will be finishing two-thirds of your pregnancy—that's big! You can end this trimester with the fabulous news that the little nugget in your partner's tummy can recognize voices. So, if you have been talking to your kid often, then there's a high likelihood that it will turn to your voice even after it comes out.

Your Baby's Growth

Again, this week is just more of what already is. The baby, by now, can very well taste the difference between whatever the mother chooses to eat. For instance, if the mother has some spicy sriracha meatballs, the baby will feel the kick too and may start hiccuping in response to the taste of the amniotic fluid.

By this week, (if you can locate it,) you might even be able to hear the heartbeat by pressing your ear to the mother's belly. This signifies that the heartbeat is strong and growing and the baby is big enough so that there's no need for a Doppler or ultrasound or even a stethoscope.

Your Partner's Experience

Around this time your partner may complain of heat rashes and reddening of palms and soles. These can even be unpleasantly itchy. The overall skin complaints may be on the rise as the due date draws closer.

The clumsiness as a result of a changed center of gravity may continue along with all the pregnancy brain symptoms. Carpal tunnel syndrome might persist with backaches, leg spasms, and so on.

What You Can Do

If you and your partner are leaning towards a doula, then it might be time to get into the action, interviewing candidates to find someone who is a perfect match.

As for the rashes and redness, remind your partner to avoid situations that cause more redness and heat like tight gloves and clothes. Ice packs and frozen fruit can be simple remedies that bring great relief for her. Itchiness can be soothed by lotion or even some coconut oil, whichever she prefers.

While workout remains crucial, make sure you remind your partner not to overexert herself. A talk test might be a hassle-free way of making sure she doesn't strain her and the baby's heart too much—if she can't talk when she is working out, it's probably overworking her heart.

And with that, you are on your final lap! Start practicing that victory dance, you'll need to break out the moves soon enough!

8

THE SEVENTH MONTH

"It's the final countdown!" That's the song playing in your head all the time now—when you're slicing that knife through those tomatoes, when you're driving that cart dangerously through the supermarket aisle picking up the best diapers from the shelf, and when you are dripping with bright happy colors as you paint the nursery! Yup, you are the dude dad and the final trimester will surely make you feel like it.

THE WEEK-BY-WEEK PROGRESS

In the last chapter, we mentioned viability and the survival chances of the baby being somewhere between 50 to 75%. Now—brace yourself because this is big news—the baby's survival rate jumps to the late 90s depending on which week the baby is born. Now those are some really good odds and that means a massive drop in the anxiety about the baby's well-being in your as well as your partner's head. But don't get too attached to that peace of mind because it will soon be replaced by the anxiety of doing things right when the baby arrives.

Week 28

By this time the baby is preparing for birth by moving into a head-down position which is crucial for a smooth delivery in a couple of months. If your partner has still been doing all those big and small chores around the house, it's time to put on your game face buddy!

Your Baby's Growth

With other organs fairly in place, the brain is working in top gear. The lungs are strengthening by the day too. Around this time, the baby is showing signs of rapid eye movement sleep aka the REM sleep and is very likely to be dreaming. The baby is also putting to good use the eyelashes and the eyelids that it has developed by batting them open and shut.

During this week, it is often observed that the baby is sticking out its tongue as if making faces. However, this is more likely its attempt to taste the amniotic fluid.

Overall the baby is now the average size of an eggplant and weighs over two pounds. From the head of a pin to begin with to an eggplant, your baby, your partner and you have taken on a long, adventurous journey.

Your Partner's Experience

Sciatic pain is a common occurrence in mothers at this stage. This is primarily because the baby is exerting more and more pressure on the sciatic nerve. As the growing baby presses upwards against her lungs, it is likely to impact her own lung capacity leading to shortness of breath. Not to forget the kicks and punches that are getting all too frequent and strong! These can cause discomfort at best and can be painful at worst.

What You Can Do

You'll need to keep track of the increased frequency of the third-trimester check-ups. While till now they have been scheduled every four weeks, from now on, they will be scheduled every two weeks so that the mother's and the baby's vitals can be monitored more closely. Your partner might also be advised to do an Rh test, which if negative, might require her to take immunoglobulin injections.

Yoga can also help her relieve her aching body. If you haven't yet, break into those yoga pants you got months ago and get to work as you support her body when she is doing poses like the pigeon pose. Make sure that these poses are done with proper guidance and under expert supervision. You don't want your partner to over-stretch herself. Literally.

As the third trimester begins, the baby is using up all of its iron reserves and therefore the Mommy must get a fair amount of iron through her diet. Foods like spinach, dates, dried apricots, raspberries, etc. can help avoid complications like anemia.

Week 29

The baby is quite close to average birth height and is close to 16 inches long. It's now a good three pounds in weight. A good idea right about now would be to find a pediatrician that you love. Yes, love! That is a person you are going to be visiting quite often and you have got to make sure you, your partner, and your doctor (and later possibly even your baby) are on the same page.

Your Baby's Growth

One thing that is sure to get those "Awww"s is the baby is now smiling in its sleep. No, it's not the social smile we are all used to. Smiling probably means that it is only passing gas. The baby does not understand the complex emotion of joy when it is flatulent. Or does it?

The baby's skeleton is also hardening at this point. The bones are being deposited with almost 200 mg of Calcium every day. The baby's forehead is developed by now but is quite uneven and bulging because of the growing brain. Yup, something like the Martians from "Mars Attack!", just cuter and with skin! This will change in the coming weeks but for now, the focus is on the rest of the body. It's hello fatty tissue and bye-bye wrinkles. The baby is going to get fatter over the next couple of months until it comes out all chubby and cute.

Your Partner's Experience

The Braxton Hicks are likely to come on much more frequently and strongly. It might get a little difficult for the mother to identify real contractions from the false alarms. It's best to consult your healthcare provider to look for the most common signs of real labor.

The mother's breasts are now tuning in to the coming pregnancy as they start getting damp from time to time from the colostrum that is produced. This is the result of the production of prolactin as the breasts gear up for a lactation phase.

What You Can Do

As time goes by your partner is going to need to use the bathroom ALL the time. So, ensure that she has access to a bathroom wherever she goes. It might feel like a quick chore for you but her bladder may not think that.

As the breasts get wet on random occasions, breast pads are a worthy purchase to avoid embarrassing situations in public. It's also always a great idea to keep a change of clothes or a jacket with you wherever she goes.

Her restless leg syndrome might be beginning to grow worse in this trimester. Make sure she is getting some exercise even though it gets difficult for her.

Now, you can also think of enrolling in childbirth classes. Do not miss out on these because this is likely to help you bond over the baby in a very real manner.

Week 30

This week your partner's belly is ballooned up even more as the baby is rapidly gaining fats. The discomfort is nowhere even near over for your partner and will only get worse until the baby exits.

Your Baby's Growth

The brain is developing at a swift pace. It is getting wrinkly and will develop the grooves and fissures that provide for more surface area for the growth of brain cells. As the fats depositing under the baby's skin regulate its temperature, the fine hair growth called lanugo that appeared a while back to keep it warm, is now disappearing. Most of the time, this growth has disappeared by the time the baby is born. Even if it hasn't, it will shed off soon after. The baby's bone marrow is now also producing red blood cells.

Your Partner's Experience

The ligaments that began relaxing sometime back are relaxing further to aid the pregnancy process. The tender breasts have returned with a vengeance as they prepare for breastfeeding. Of course, not everyone will have the same experience and who knows, you and your partner might be among the few who feel pretty great even through this week.

What You Can Do

Your doctor might screen your partner for staph infection as this can be transmitted to the baby through the milk. They might also recommend what's known as a kick count test to make sure the baby's vitals are good. Here, the mother would count the number of kicks, punches, rolls, flutters, and all other movements per hour. If this number is less than ten for two hours, it might be best to call your healthcare provider. You can use the tips I gave you earlier to induce this kicking—grab a snack for your partner and let her lie down.

Now would be the perfect time to do a detailed survey of your home to figure out the things that would require baby-proofing, for instance, electricity outlets, any cleaning chemicals, any sharp or glass objects, and so on. You need to make a list and follow some baby-proofing guides if needed.

Week 31

Wow! You have made it to the home stretch! After this week it will only be nine more weeks. Take some time out and appreciate how far you have come because in a few more weeks you won't have much spare time for things like appreciation. Think of that moment when you and your partner held that stick. Even though you wanted to be a father, there was, of course, some anxiety and doubt. But somewhere along the way you have become a father even though you are yet to hold your baby in your arms. Now, that's a journey you can be proud of.

Your Baby's Growth

Okay, back to business. This week your baby is still gaining in fats and is somewhere around three to four pounds in weight. As the brain gets stronger, the baby's perceptive power from all five senses is also heightened. The kicks and punches are no cuter and can be strong enough to enter the list of things that are keeping your partner awake at night. A new development is that side-to-side head movement as the baby gains more control over its muscles.

Your Partner's Experience

By now, based on the activity, your partner is well aware of the baby's nap times and might want to nap at the same time. Fortunately, the baby is now sleeping a little more; that is the only silver lining to the dark cloud of constant discomforts your partner is experiencing.

Your partner may also start experiencing something known as the lightning crotch. Sure, laugh it off! Take it out of your system and then never make fun of it in front of your partner. As funny as it sounds, it can also be quite painful as she may experience a shooting pain like an electrical bolt or shock in the vagina, pelvis, or even rectum. The possible reason for this is that the baby is now pressing on a nerve leading to the cervix.

What You Can Do

The pain she is experiencing might be alleviated by warm baths, changing positions, and even wearing a support band. As you get busy with cooking meals and filling up your freezer, it might also be a good time to plan babycare once it arrives. You might want to discuss things like who will get up in the middle of the night when the baby starts crying. In the case that you both cannot do it, you might have to think of hiring someone to do it for the baby. This may seem detached but remember that parenting is not about draining yourself to the point that you cannot function at all. Practical, innovative solutions are also a major part of parenting. So, go ahead, talk about it and have a plan ready.

With only nine more weeks to go, it all might seem like a lot to take in. But remember that your partner has done the heavy lifting in this stretch, after the baby arrives, it'll be your turn. And if you have stuck through this book for so long rather than switching on ESPN then it means you are in it for real and you'll be just fine!

9

THE EIGHTH MONTH

One more month to go after this. Yes, at the end of this month you'll have a mere five weeks, if at all until the baby arrives.

THE WEEK-BY-WEEK PROGRESS

Depending on the symptoms that your partner has been experiencing, you might either find time to revel in this fact or you might just want to be done with it! Either way, it is going to be over pretty soon. So, pull on that seatbelt because the ride is not over yet!

Week 32

With the due date approaching, it's quite common for the mother to get cranky and irritated as sleep becomes a rare commodity for her. The need to pee is now constant with the baby squishing up her bladder (and other organs) more and more. The heartburn might be getting worse by the day too.

Your Baby's Growth

The baby is now closing in on four pounds and is around 17 inches long. The lungs are the last organ to develop as they are still practicing breathing skills by inhaling and exhaling the amniotic fluid.

Your baby now has opaque skin and all its organs except for lungs are fully formed. If by chance, your partner goes into early labor now, the baby would still be A-okay barring any other complications. The baby also realizes it's almost time and might move to the lower part of the uterus.

Your Partner's Experience

As her belly keeps increasing in size, you are likely to have heard the word fundal height thrown around at your medical check-ups. This is nothing but the distance between the pubic bone to the top of the uterus. As time goes by, this obviously increases and this week it's somewhere around 13 inches.

Braxton Hicks contractions are growing stronger and more frequent. Your partner, by now, knows that actual labor contractions are different in that they gradually increase in strength and occur closer together, and disappear when she changes position. The dampening of breasts continues and is here to stay until even after birth.

What You Can Do

Now is the time to bring your healthcare provider in on the birth plan that you and your partner have discussed and finalized. You and her doula would, of course, be there to support her through the birth in the delivery room, but all of you must be on the same page right from the start. When discussing the plan with your partner, it would also be a good idea to have a backup. But if you and your partner feel strongly about something don't hesitate to let the healthcare team know.

On a more fun note, this is probably the time your partner's close friends or family are planning a baby shower for the Mommy-to-be. If they want you in on the planning of the surprise, be a team player and enjoy the fun. It's a deeply fulfilling moment to see your partner, who has been going through too many hardships, crack a smile, kick back, and relax.

Week 33

By now the baby has reached its full length but the fat deposition is still a work in progress. It is putting on almost half a pound each week. Needless to say, your partner's belly is also gaining in inches fast.

Your Baby's Growth

The baby's immune system is also in place now as the antibodies from the mother travel to the baby. Though all of the baby's organs are quite well-developed at this stage, there is still one crucial part of the baby's body that is still quite vulnerable—the skull. The skeletal plates in the skull have not fully fused, thus leaving a soft spot known as the fontanel. This isn't by mistake but rather by design. This pliable head will make the baby's journey through the birth canal and finally squeezing out of the vagina far easier than if it was a hard skull.

Your Partner's Experience

This month your partner is likely to have pregnancy dreams. Yes, even the little sleep she is sneaking in is often riddled with highly realistic dreams and night-mares that mothers remember even after waking up. This is usually due to the intense stress the mother is going through physically and emotionally. She must be able to talk about this because they can trigger some quite intense emotions including feelings of guilt for dreaming something ominous about the baby or even you, the father. This means you might be apologizing for cheating on her, even if it did only happen in her dream.

What You Can Do

Go over the details with the hospital or the birthing center you have registered at. Make sure you have a room that can be shared with your baby at all times. While you are at the hospital discussion, also talk about who you would want in the hospital and also in the delivery room with you. More people around isn't always something you and your partner would be comfortable with. The staph results will also be back by now; make sure you factor this into the breastfeeding decision.

A simple yet fulfilling thing is to record a message of some sort for your baby. Share your utmost happiness and hopes for this little bundle of joy that's going to change your life forever. Maybe they can view/read the message someday in the future, a time capsule of their own.

Week 34

At five pounds this week, the baby is getting quite heavy to carry. Can you believe that the mom's uterus is now anywhere between 500 to 1000 times bigger than it was before pregnancy? You can be sure that by now she misses seeing her toes and hopes to do it soon enough.

Your Baby's Growth

If it's a boy the testicles have fully come down and are housed in the scrotum which is also fully developed. This, however, doesn't always happen and some boys have their testicles drop down even a year after birth.

The baby's lungs are almost at the finish line and will be fully developed by the end of this week. The baby's size is now similar to cantaloupe and its head is steadily moving downward toward the pelvis.

Your Partner's Experience

The discomforts of pregnancy are only getting worse and with her constant urination, she runs the risk of getting dehydrated if she does not take in enough fluids. As the end comes within sight, she is likely to start worrying over how everything will go.

What You Can Do

One thing to know here is that no matter how much you plan ahead, those plans will still go south for some completely unexpected reason. Know that it's okay, and you didn't necessarily do anything wrong. The only way to do this is to keep thinking of backups and pray with all your heart that one of them works out. Make sure you know the fastest and the slowest routes to your hospital. Once your partner goes into labor, it's going to be panic central in there! Don't wait till the last moment to figure out the logistics of how you'll get there.

Make sure your car seat is strapped and ready to go; you never know, with the next drive you might be bringing home that baby you ordered!

Week 35

This week the much-awaited lung development is through and if it comes out now, the baby would be able to breathe on its own. The other organs are also fully developed by now. The only things that will continue this week are weight gain and brain development.

Your Baby's Growth

As the space in Mommy's uterus becomes more and more restricted for the growing baby, the kicks and punches are likely to subside and be replaced with wiggles and flutters. At this point, the majority of your baby's development is in terms of gaining fat.

Your Partner's Experience

Until a few days ago, the baby was pushing on one side against the lungs causing shortness of breath, and on the other side against the bladder causing frequent urination. Once the baby moves downward in the uterus, your partner's lungs might feel relief but the baby now has an exclusive pass to her bladder. This can even lead to urinary incontinence but come what may, you need to encourage your partner to keep drinking fluids.

What You Can Do

As miserable as your partner is feeling right now, you need to be her cheerleader. Encourage her to hit the gym whenever she can because her exercise might just help the newborn when it arrives sleep through the night much quicker than otherwise.

If you haven't already, consider this your final warning! Pack that hospital bag because there is no way around it now! You will likely be getting to drive to the hospital any time now and you must be ready at least in terms of your wardrobe.

The baby can come anytime now, so get in the zone bro! No more time to waste!

10

THE NINTH MONTH

P inch yourself because it's real. You are finally here. The final few weeks before you can hold your baby. All that you and your partner have gone through will finally feel like it's worth it. But you still have a few weeks to go before you revel in the joy (or frustrations) of becoming a parent.

This is your last chance to wrap up all your work and home projects before you make the trip to the hospital. It's, of course, not like you are going to the land of no return but remember when you come back you'll have a full-fledged, hungry, crying, and (hopefully not) a colicky baby. You'll probably end up spending a lot of your time soothing, feeding, or just plain staring at the marvel you have created. Long story short, you will not find the time to wrap up those incomplete projects for a while, at least until you figure out your schedule.

So, this is the last call dude! Finish up the baby proofing tasks that you have procrastinated on till now, get the nursery to look as cozy as you can complete with a rocking chair, and pack that diaper bag already!

THE WEEK-BY-WEEK PROGRESS

Your partner is quite likely going to be just as cranky as the baby when it gets hungry. And honestly, she is doing her part of carrying that sugar bag around for you. So, get in there and do whatever you can do before she feels compelled to do it. That will be a win you can carry around proudly.

Week 36

The baby is now almost fully developed and is around 19 inches long and getting heavier at a solid six pounds. The weight-gaining still hasn't gotten old and continues at a brisk pace.

Your Baby's Growth

This week your baby starts looking like the cute self that it will be when it comes out as the cheeks are filling out with fat. As it gets bigger the movements become more crammed in and are thus not as noticeable as before. The digestive system is fully developed. Your baby hasn't been exposed to milk yet but is producing dark green waste called meconium by digesting the amniotic fluid. Not much else is happening, except for the baby practicing all of the survival functions that it will be required to perform the moment it leaves the comfort of the womb. The circulatory and skeletal systems are functioning as they should by now. Overall, the baby just seems to be chilling.

Your Partner's Experience

If this is her first pregnancy, the baby is likely to drop further towards the pelvis this week. This is often referred to as lightening. The swelling and back pains continue and the connective tissue, muscles, and ligaments continue to loosen up in anticipation of the delivery.

What You Can Do

Now the appointments will happen in high gear as your partner will be scheduled for a checkup every week. Try to make these visits with your partner because sometimes a complicated position of the child that comes up during one of these visits can get overwhelming for your partner.

Continue encouraging her to relax with her feet elevated to alleviate the swelling. It is also the time that your partner will stop all air travel because it isn't considered to be safe or any kind of travel really, because she just may not be in a mood to carry the burgeoning belly anywhere other than she has to.

Week 37

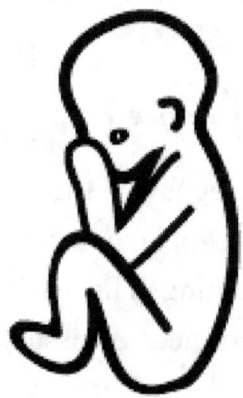

This week marks the end of preterm or early-term deliveries. That means if the baby is born this week it will be considered a full-term baby.

Your Baby's Growth

The baby continues its half a pound per week weight gain streak. By now it's about six and a half pounds. It's only killing time in the womb by moving from side to side and taking in the amniotic fluid. There aren't many other changes happening at this point except that it might continue to drop further on its exit path.

Your Partner's Experience

A sudden reemergence of the nesting energy that made an appearance earlier might be hard to miss in your partner. She is as uncomfortable as ever and she still will make you move things around over and over until it seems perfect to her. Believe me, you don't want to fight her on this. The mother instinct is hard at play here and you don't want to mess with that! And generally, that instinct is quite right.

What You Can Do

The doctor might do a physical evaluation of the cervix to gauge how things are going. This is usually an exciting time for couples and you shouldn't miss it if possible.

This might even be a good time to look for a pelvic floor therapist and enquire about a perineal massage. Don't worry, no one is overtaking your position but getting a trained professional to massage the area between your partner's vagina and rectal area can help stretch the skin and may even help avoid tearing and the episiotomy procedure.

As her heartburn increases you may have to sit her down and make her eat those small meals you have been planning so intently. Accompany her to do her stretches on that exercise ball. You also want to do a final sweep of anything that may have been left behind from your plan and make sure everything is in place.

Week 38

The baby is now almost seven pounds this week. And though technically there are still a couple more weeks to go, the baby is ready for the world. If the baby is ready, it wouldn't be too far-fetched to say that the mother is more than ready for the baby to come out. But both of you might already be thinking of the future battle.

Your Baby's Growth

The vocal cord development that started a while back is now finally completed this week. That means that along with the lungs it has developed the baby will be able to give a full-throated wailing cry when it comes out. That in itself is a big indicator that all is well.

Your Partner's Experience

The lightening process continues as the baby moves further down in the pelvis. This leads to the cervix softening and the cervical opening dilating to allow for the passage of the baby. The mother cannot dream of going anywhere without knowing where the bathroom is.

What You Can Do

The baby's position is of utmost importance to your birthing plan. If at this stage one of the ultrasounds reveals the baby to be in a breech position, you will have to give up on that birthing plan of yours as the doctor will likely schedule a C-section. It's crucial to know at this point that even though you have spent a long time planning for this, nothing always goes according to plan.

If a C-section can be avoided then you might want to help your partner research techniques that can help her get through labor. If you have a doula, this will be her job. Encourage her to plan workouts that have squats reps as these facilitate pelvic opening

Week 39

The delivery can happen any moment now! Though the due date isn't until the 40th week, babies are rarely born on the calculated date.

Your Baby's Growth

The baby is shedding its skin along with the lanugo and new skin is taking its place. This skin is less pink and more whitish or greyish. Though the baby has formed tear ducts, they won't open until about a month after birth. The baby is now almost as big as honeydew melon and weighs almost about eight pounds. The baby continues brain development and gains weight. But apart from these two, further development is halted until delivery.

Your Partner's Experience

You can be sure that your partner's discomforts aren't going anywhere until the baby arrives. But even through these, she will likely be alert to any symptoms of labor like the amniotic sac rupturing, often known as water breaking, the falling off of the mucus plug that covers the uterine opening, and so on.

What You Can Do

There isn't much you can do at this point other than making sure your partner is as comfortable as she can be. Get those essential oils out (only the ones that are okay for use during pregnancy) and let her enjoy some pleasant fragrances, some soothing music, and a nice warm bath. Before you know it, any spare time for her and you will be a distant dream.

Week 40

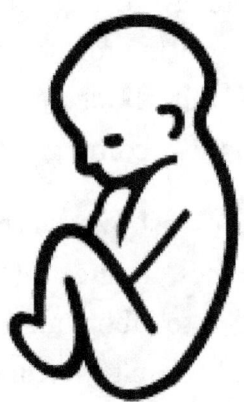

This is it! The official end of your pregnancy. If the baby still hasn't arrived, your partner is likely beyond exhausted as well as irritated. While the mother, as well as the baby, are biologically perfectly ready for the delivery, the baby just may not be in a mood to come down. Your healthcare provider, at this point, may discuss the idea of induced labor, either through some natural remedies like spicy food or sex, or medicated inducement.

Your Baby's Growth

The baby's weight might not be known for certain until it goes out of the birth canal and onto the weighing scale.

Your Partner's Experience

Your partner is likely going through a massive emotional upheaval waiting for her cervix to dilate. Just as you are freaking out about becoming a dad, she is also freaking out about becoming a mom.

Remember that labor is one of the most painfully exhausting experiences in life. Of course, I have no experience in going into labor but I have seen my wife go through it and it doesn't look like a spa treatment. Be sure to be empathetic to the anxieties as well as the pain. When in labor she will first expel the baby and then the placenta.

What You Can Do

Be reachable ALL the time, the call can come any moment. Make sure your partner has all that she needs when in the delivery room. It's now time to put all those birthing classes to great use.

NO BABY STILL?

It so happens that a considerable percentage of babies are born in the 41st and the 42nd weeks too! This can be especially difficult and may even feel anticlimactic to the mother. The baby isn't considered post-term until after the 42nd week but it's unlikely that your health-care provider would wait that long.

Whatever the case, the most important thing is to not let this get to you and your partner. Remember that many times what feels like a post-term delivery might simply be a miscalculated pregnancy date.

Take this extra time to finish up on whatever necessary tasks you might have left hanging. Be clear about your paternity leave policy and try to use it as wisely as possible. If after all birth is through a C-section, you might find it much easier to plan out your leave because the uncertainty can be finally lifted. But the demerit of C-section is the longer recovery times which might anyway require you to be around for long.

Through all this, while your partner and baby are your focus, don't forget to take some time out for yourself. Be it watching a stress-free game of football or going for a drive to clear out your mind or even just a simple workout by yourself, your downtime is crucial to keep yourself as well as your partner in a hopeful state of mind despite the anxieties regarding the reasons for the possible delayed birth. Take this time to go over your childbirth class techniques with your partner. That is likely to keep your eyes on the prize and steer you away from the frustration at least in a small way.

11

BRINGING HOME THE BABY— THE FIRST MONTH

There you go! A full-fledged human baby, and that too your own! I bet you never thought you could do this. But you have and you get to take home the trophy to prove your win strapped into the backseat of your car! You have done well because you have done all you could.

But if you thought the difficult part was over, then oh boy, you are getting burnt and how! Now that the pregnancy battle has been won with your partner on the frontline, it's time to get to the next battle—getting the baby home and caring for it.

Most people think that once you get home from the hospital, it's back to life as you have always known it. Well, these people have most probably never been through this whole process. The truth is the mother's body requires at least a month to cope with all that she has been through, not just physically but also emotionally. And as much as Superdad may want to sweep in and save the day, remember that you have been through a rollercoaster of your own too.

So, take a step back and don't be in a hurry to set the routine yet. Soak in your partner's and the baby's presence and make sure you meet the baby's needs. The rest of the routine will fall in place.

DIVIDE AND CONQUER

The best way to keep your sanity through being a new parent is to divide the responsibilities. You have likely already discussed this with your partner. But revisit the conversation. What is your schedule like? Can you divide the midnight feeding and changing responsibilities on alternate days? Or if you have a hectic work schedule can you handle the weekends? At least a few hours of uninterrupted sleep is extremely important for both of you. If the Mommy is too tired and you are too busy, getting a night nurse or a doula might be a great alternative.

A doula will not only take care of the baby but also pay attention to the nutrition of the baby, share healthy recipes and overall provide your partner with substantial physical and emotional support. But this great option also has a cost.

While it may seem tempting because of the convenience it offers, remember that getting someone to care for your baby simply means you don't get to do it. I'm just stating the obvious, I know but I can tell you from my experience that I would never give up on those moments that I shared with my newborn, no matter how difficult they might have seemed. These are the moments that you get to develop your own equation with your child right from the beginning.

Taking care of that tiny thing (your partner surely didn't think that when it came out of her) is one of the most rewarding experiences you will have. It may include seemingly trivial tasks like bathing, changing diapers, soothing when crying, etc. But the truth is these give a much-needed opportunity to establish physical contact with the father. The bonus is it helps establish some sort of symmetrical distribution of responsibilities amongst you and your partner. But while fulfilling these responsibilities don't forget to have fun. Ensure that you keep talking and singing to the baby. If you did it before the delivery, the baby probably recognizes your voice. That can be a great boost for your relationship.

A FEW HOW TO'S TO SAVE YOUR LIFE

I have often observed that men do not proactively participate in childcare for the fear that they might somehow screw up and break the baby. I know because I used to feel the same. But over the years I have realized it's all about blending a brilliant fun personality with a few basic skills and voila! The dude Dad is unstoppable. I believe all dads have that fun personality quite innately. As for the skills, here are a few how-tos that will save you a lot of anxiety and many fights with your partner.

All About Diapers

Changing diapers is one of the most feared tasks in the quiet streets of the Daddy community. But let me tell you a secret. It's not rocket science. It's all about getting the knack right. Here's a step-by-step standard operating procedure when it comes to mission mud butt.

1. First things first. Make sure you have all your supplies in one place. That includes wipes, diapers, petroleum jelly, and a cloth pad to place the baby on. Remember that you can never leave the baby alone even for a moment to go and get the wipes or something else that you forgot. So, it's just easier to gather

everything before you begin the climb to the diaper Everest.

2. Next, unfasten the diaper, lift the baby gently by its ankles, and dispose of the evidence. Make sure to wipe the baby from front to back. Doing it in the opposite direction may result in the spreading of bacteria from the anal region thereby leading to UTIs especially among girls.

3. There are various diapers available on the market. If you are using a disposable one, you will first open it and put it under the baby. Gently raise the baby's legs and slide them underneath. Keep the strips from the back part somewhat level with the baby's belly button. Then cover the baby's front with the front part of the diaper and fasten the adhesive tapes. Don't stick the tape to the baby.

Easy enough? You won't know until you try. So practice because that's the only way to get it right.

The Burping Basics

Another skill that will save you a ton of anguish is learning how to burp the baby. Gas can be painful for the babies as well as for you. There are more or less three ways you can tackle this.

1. Hold the baby against your chest and let it rest its chin on your shoulder. Support the baby with one hand while you pat it on the back with the other. I find this to be easier than the other techniques.
2. Let the baby sit on your lap across the knees. Keep one hand against the baby's chest in a way that she can rest her chin on your palm. With the other hand, pat the baby on the back.
3. Keep the baby on its belly. Make sure the head is supported and is higher than the belly and then pat the back.

Yup, it's that simple. I know that in the beginning whenever you hold the baby it will feel like you are holding a million-dollar (maybe even more), fragile crystal glass as if the slightest misstep will break the baby. While a few basic things need to be kept in mind, remember your baby is not as fragile as it looks. That is one resilient creature. You definitely should be careful as to how you handle the baby but don't let that feeling instill fear of getting close to it.

The Bathing Stories

If your baby has had circumcision, it's best not to bathe the baby until that heals, which is around the first two weeks. Also, keep in mind that the umbilical cord needs to fall off and the belly button needs to be completely healed. Either way, for the first couple of weeks it's going to be a sponge bath for your little pumpkin.

Sponge baths may seem like a breeze and they usually are but be mindful of the lather not going into the baby's eyes. Use warm water, dip the washcloth with water and squeeze out the extra liquid. Gently use the cloth to wipe the baby's eyes. Pay specific attention to the nose, ears, and clean them properly.

Use a bit of soap to create lather, and wash the baby's head all the while taking care not to let the lather go into the baby's eyes. Make sure you clean the creases and crevices of your baby's butt and thighs to avoid rashes or infections.

SOME PRO-DAD QUICK TIPS

With the above three skills, you have covered quite some ground. The baby isn't the only one that should be getting pats on the back. A little earlier we spoke of how if you follow the absolute basics the baby's resilient nature will take care of the rest. In addition to the one we mentioned earlier—never leave the baby unattended—here are some more of those basics.

1. (Don't) shake it baby: The baby's muscular

control is still not great, especially when it comes to the neck. If the baby is vigorously shaken the head may go back and forth violently. This in turn may lead the brain to bang against the skull causing severe damage.

2. Wash wash wash: When handling a baby, make sure you wash your hands clean with soap for at least 15 seconds. Remember the baby's immune system is still not strong enough to ward off any infection that comes its way. And even if it is, nothing good can come out of needlessly straining that system all the time. So, if you are the kind who doesn't wash those hands after having some saucy wings, then you really shouldn't be picking up the baby.

3. Support the head: Your baby will eventually gain control over those muscles but for now it needs to be supported. Whenever you hold a baby, make sure you use one hand to support the head. As you become a pro, you will find that you can do it even with one hand.

4. Strap on the seat: Car seats can be tricky. Ensure that you have had multiple checks before you seat your precious cargo in the back. Make sure it's safe and that you have followed the manual instructions to the tee.

12

MONEY MATTERS

It's an undeniable fact that we live in crazy expensive times. Raising a child in these times is no joke and is as much a financial decision as an emotional one. When I became a dad for the first time, this was one of the first things that popped in my head, "How much was this whole thing going to cost me?" and "Where the hell am I going to get all that money from?!" The answer to the first question was "A lot!" However, the answer to the second question would have been much easier had I known where to look and what to do.

As my wife gave birth to our first child, I was as clueless as the next guy, unless the next guy was a born-to-be-dad kind of a guy! Anyway, I had to go through the trenches to learn my lesson the hard way. But now that

I know, it almost seems stupid not to have known before. Don't be the clueless father that I was the first time around. Today, I know that though the financial aspect can be intimidating, you will find that it's not that difficult to find the right answers if you ask the right questions.

BUILDING THE BABY BUDGET

If you think that you will just fling it with the finances once the baby arrives, you will find yourself in a sea of trouble in no time. Therefore, the first step is to plan ahead. Having a family isn't a decision you want to make overnight. The financial aspect needs to be in the background whenever you have conversations surrounding the baby. But also remember, just talking about it isn't enough. Acting on it at the earliest is key.

To tell you the truth, building a baby budget isn't too different from a normal budget. But the problem is most of us tend to shy away the moment we hear the word budget. Call it planning if you like but know that there is no way around it.

First off, sit down and determine your income sources. You need to track down every last penny to its source and only then can you effectively allocate it to the required expenses. Make a list of all the sources money comes from.

The next step is to determine the categories of expenses. If you are just starting out in the initial stages, and have some time to accumulate the funds, you can merely include the baby fund as a category in addition to other categories like the emergency fund, debt payment, bills, leisure, health, and so on. Most people prefer using the envelope system whereby they assign one envelope to each category and distribute every last dollar from their income to all of these categories depending on the need. So, let's say I have $1,000. I would allocate the entire amount based on the 50/30/20 rule—50% would go to my necessities like bills, groceries, health, debts, etc. 30% goes to leisure, entertainment, and things that I want but are not really necessities so to say and 20% gets divided into an emergency fund, baby fund and so on. Now, once the division is made, there's no going back. For instance, if I run out of cash in my dine-out envelope, I cannot sneak the unused money from the other envelopes. This system is often found to be effective in bringing financial discipline to even the people who complain of the rigidity of budgets.

If at all you don't have enough time, it may be recommended that you prioritize the baby fund over other things and allocate the maximum possible amount here. The baby fund can be further divided into health, accessories, necessities, gear, childcare, and so on, depending on your requirements. But note that prioritizing does not mean that you only dedicate money to the baby funds and ignore other things like toxic debt. Prioritization only means that the amount trickling into those categories will be smaller for some time.

It is also beneficial to cut down on lavish expenses for a while and live on the bare minimum possible. This is some pretty practical advice I received because you may have already lost or might soon be losing out on a chunk of one parent who goes on leave for a while. The oncoming expenses can lead to a considerable financial pinch especially if you haven't been saving for the baby.

SOME PRO-SAVER QUICK TIPS

Here are a few tips to help you become the pro-budgeteer that can help you get your head in the financial game. Of course, this isn't some great wisdom. We all know this and yet need someone else to remind us now and then.

1. Shopping lists are important: Wherever you go shopping, buy only those things that are on the list. Though this applies to even grocery

shopping, it is even more crucial when shopping for a baby. Even as the macho man that you might be, you will melt when you see Daddy's little girl or Daddy Junior onesies. Make sure you stick to buying only what's needed.

2. Coupons are lifesavers: If you were ever too fancy to use coupons, as a parent those days are behind you. You have to save whatever you can and if coupons let you do it, so be it!

3. Bargaining is a parenting skill too: As your child grows up, you will be frequently required to negotiate. Consider this practice for your future. Bargain wherever you can. Ask for loyalty discounts if you frequent the place often. Whatever saves you the extra buck is worth it.

4. Shop around: We as men are wired to buy the first thing that suits our needs without making a fuss. Well, now that you have a fussy baby you can't avoid it anymore. Shop around for the best price that you can get. Whether it's insurance, a car seat, or any other service, make sure you check out a few competitors in the category and then make an informed and economical decision.

5. Debt is a no-no: The only debt that might do

you some good is your mortgage. If possible, you can even think about refinancing your mortgage. Do not pile up on any other kind of debt, especially credit card debt.

13

YOUR CHANGING RELATIONSHIP

L et's cut to the chase, shall we? If anyone tells you pregnancy does not change a marriage, they are lying. That's the simple truth of it. But why is that always assumed to be a bad thing? I am not going to gloss over it and tell you that it's all rainbows and roses, nothing ever is. But here's the way I look at it. Even before the pregnancy, my relationship with my wife didn't just fall into place like a cheesy romcom. We had to work through our relationship and its ups and downs and I am pretty certain you have had to work through yours too.

But yes, pregnancy is a never-before-experienced relationship hurdle for first-time parents and can pack quite the sucker punch for those that are not ready for it. But, if you go in with a realistic perception of the process, you might be much better at dealing with whatever the pregnancy throws your way.

A TIDE OF CHANGE

Let's try something. Close your eyes for a moment, take a deep breath and think about what you expect to change in your relationship after the pregnancy. If sex was the first thing that you thought of, you got a part of it right but there is more to it than just that.

As you have seen, through the persisting symptoms that your partner has to endure, it shouldn't be a surprise that you may find your sex life slowing down quite a bit, if it moves at all, that is. It is at this point that the difference between sex and intimacy might become quite apparent to the two of you. Though the partner may not be up for sex, she may not mind romance at all. And the thing with romance, as you know, needs history, unlike the act of sex.

If you want to keep the romantic spark alive during pregnancy, you will have to find ways to reconnect with each other much before her pregnancy queasiness starts. Take her on a surprise date every once in a while. Bring home her favorite treats. Remember that relationships are reciprocal, what goes around will surely come around. Also, it's interesting to note that sex is never really out of bounds during pregnancy unless your partner is at risk, as in the case of pre-term or multiple births. So, if you can get her engine going, it won't take too long to get things hot and steamy.

So, now that the sex part is sorted, what else could impact the relationship? Well, unfortunately, the sex problem might just have the most straightforward solution. Another pregnancy aspect that might make your relationship bumpy is the fact that your partner's raging hormones are likely to make her clingy. Many women express fears of abandonment when pregnant. This may be due to her changing body or simply the uncertainties of things to come. But whatever it is, these fears, if left unaddressed, can pile up to be explosive for your relationship.

Open communication is paramount to this dynamic. Be an active listener to your partner. The important thing is to validate each other's psychological experiences rather than discarding them or even frowning at them. Remember your body language says a lot more than your words. Show them openness through your gestures, facial expressions, and tone. Only when you reassure her through your actions, will her fears be allayed. And even if they don't, remember the insecurity is temporary.

Another reason for this changing relationship is the difference in perspectives. As the pregnancy comes on, your partner may feel frustrated about the lack of involvement from your side, even when you are trying your best. In reality, the difference is that while the pregnancy is real for her right from the third or the fourth week, you may not experience the same immediacy until a little later.

I remember this argument coming up a lot when my wife was pregnant the first time. She would get upset that I wasn't paying attention and I didn't even know what it was that I was supposed to pay attention to. The whole purpose of this book is to create that immediacy within the first-time fathers. But, of course, you might not find it in the very beginning even after reading this book. If you ask me, fake it till you make it is the mantra to live by.

But hey like I said, the pregnancy impact doesn't always have to be negative. The pregnancy will bring you much closer to your partner than before. Believe me, when your partner can let a strong one rip as casually as ever while you are chilling with your favorite series and you end up laughing it off, you just have one more reason to love that series! The intimacy will be taken to another level once you share these moments.

So, no, your relationship won't be the same ever because you have taken it many notches higher on the comfort level. It will take some getting used to. But it's all worth it!

SOME PRO-PARTNER QUICK TIPS

Here are a few ideas to spark up that love and passion all over again. Remember it's right there buried beneath the pregnancy symptoms, responsibilities, and anxieties. It might take some special effort to rekindle it in the midst of all that's going on but if you never try, you'll never know.

1. Love on post-its: Sometimes, you don't need anything grand, all that's required is simple, honest gestures. When was the last time you told her explicitly how much you love her? Try doing it now, leave her post-its in random unexpected places and see that frown turn upside down.

2. Surprise dates: Remember the time you used to date, how exciting it was? Awaken that excitement by doing something completely spontaneous. Take her someplace nice with music and her favorite food or stay in and binge on some shows or movies. Just make her feel

special and you'll notice those insecurities melting away. For her, intimacy at this stage may not always mean physical intimacy; cuddling (if her breasts haven't gotten sore yet), kissing, and even holding hands may serve the purpose of bringing you closer together.

3. Spice it up: Send her a random sexy text and carry on the conversation for a bit. Give her those foot and back massages, light some aromatic candles and see where the night takes you. Remember though that both of you need to be on the same page to enjoy this.

4. Active listening: You won't believe this but active listening can be a major turn-on for your partner. As mentioned above, listen with your body, and listen more than you talk. Avoid giving solutions to the problems unless she specifically asks you for them but ask her about her day, about what her hopes and dreams are for the baby, about the changes the baby will bring into their lives, and so on. Paraphrase what they have said back to them to tell them you understand their situation or at least that you're trying. This will relieve a lot of stress between you two.

5. Communicating discontent the right way: Keeping the romance alive does not mean you

cannot disagree with each other. But when you do, make sure you focus on the problem and its solution rather than blaming each other. Be sure to use "I" statements such as "I feel hurt by this." rather than saying "You have hurt me." In this phase of life, your patience will bear priceless fruit. So, have patience with her as the pregnancy hormones give rise to brain fog and make her judgments and perceptions sometimes off the track.

14

TAKING CARE OF YOURSELF

How many times in the last few months have you asked yourself what you want? Well, very likely, you haven't. This is not because you are a selfless saint but because the past few months have been all about either your partner or the baby inside her. And it's quite possible that between work, household chores, your partner, and the baby, you have not particularly paid attention to your own physical and mental health.

Sure, the battles that we, as men, fight may not be as intense as the ones your partner is fighting through her pregnancy. But it is important not to trivialize your own health too. Right now you are the behind-the-scenes guy. Think of an animated movie. Your partner and the baby are the lead character voiceovers who are of course very important but you are the sound engineer who makes those brilliant voices shine. Not many people would know the person who has designed the sound for their favorite movie but they know the leads. That's just how it is. But without your support and encouragement, the mother would find it tremendously difficult to get to this point. Therefore you need to take some downtime to yourself and do something relaxing.

THE BURDEN OF FATHERHOOD

Men have been raised to not talk about their feelings. "Crying like a girl," they say! From my own experiences and those of other men around me, I can confidently say this attitude has done more harm than good. When we lost our baby, though no one said it to me, I felt this intense internal compulsion to "man up" and move on. It was later when I revisited that experience and unleashed those repressed feelings that I saw what a ridiculous idea our society has of manhood.

The one thing I learned from the experience of that miscarriage was to seek help when needed. Ask and many will come forward to help. But the important thing is to ask. Your feelings, anxieties, self-doubt, are all just as important as your partner's. Quite a few men never put it out there on the table for the fear of being judged as "weak" or "cissy" and it all usually comes out in quite self-harming behaviors.

One such emotion I see far too often in men is the perception of being isolated. The closeness that their partner shares with their baby is upsetting to them because they feel left out which again leads to guilt creating a vicious cycle of negativity. I think most of us have been there, done that at some point in time. But now is the time to snap out of it. The only way to not be left out is to be present as much as you can. The skin-to-skin contact of the baby with the father's chest also helps in cementing this bond.

Find a support system, other than your partner. As much as you will have an open and honest communication channel, you might also have to put on a brave face for her when she is in panic mode. At this time you will need another person or people to lean on. Dads who have already been through similar situations might help just by telling you that you are not a selfish, cruel dad. They also get jealous of the way the baby sleeps peacefully in their partner's arms and starts crying bloody murder the moment they take them on. This, like all relationships, takes time to establish and you have to stop being so hard on yourself. Contrary to what you have believed all your life, talking about these feelings to someone who listens to you without judgment, helps.

One thing to definitely watch out for is signs and symptoms of depression including changes in appetite, changes in sleep pattern (that may not have much to do with the baby), irritability, total helplessness, and so on. If you find these persisting I urge you to get help.

SOME PRO-SELF-HELPER QUICK TIPS

This might seem harsh but you are useless to your partner and your baby if you are not of a sound mind and happy heart. You are their pillar of support and more importantly, now that you have experienced this beautiful miracle called life itself, there is no reason that your head should breed any self-harming negativity. Try these few self-care tips and assess the impact they bring in your life.

1. Mindful living: Mindfulness as backed by several research studies has been shown to improve people's psychological wellbeing. Note that mindfulness isn't only related to mindful meditation. Rather mindful living has more to do with being present in the current moment. I could be taking a walk and all my mental resources are focused on that one present

moment rather than thinking about something from the past or future. This may seem too hippy-dippy for you but try it once before discarding it. Every time your mind wanders you gently bring it back without any judgment.

2. Sweat the negativity out: Make sure you keep your workout schedule intact. If you have been accompanying your partner for light workouts, continue those but make it a point to finish up your own sessions also. Exercise as we know releases endorphins which biologically turn the situation in your favor.

3. Ditch the toxic masculinity: The lines between masculine and feminine are now much more blurred than before. Don't let the ancient stereotypes bring you down. Consciously remind yourself to discard those.

4. The REST formula: REST is an acronym for you to remember to take care of yourself. R for rest, E for eating, S for Support, and T for taking your time. You can be sure to improve the quality of life for yourself and consequently for your partner and the baby too.

5. Enjoy the moment: This feeling of becoming a first-time father isn't ever coming back. Sure, the joy of consequent pregnancies is there but you cannot let this first-time feeling pass by.

Also, don't be a bystander, participate in as much action as possible. If your schedule allows it, go out for a beer, if you have a no-drinking pact with your partner, no worries you can just pick up a non-alcoholic beer.

CONCLUSION

You began this journey as a complete novice who had no idea how to go through a pregnancy. Fatherhood probably turned out to be much more work than you had previously anticipated. But I guarantee you that even though it may seem a little rough in the beginning, getting pregnant is the best decision you'll make in your entire life.

We have been wired to reproduce. It keeps our species from becoming extinct after all. But what is it that makes you a Dad? Is it when you see those double lines on that plastic stick? Is it when you hold the baby in your arms? Or is it when you decide that you'll be one? Believe it or not, you have been on the path to becoming a Dad long before your partner gave birth. I believe that though we have extensively focused on the process here, the biological details have very little to do with making you feel like a father.

Reproduction has psychological benefits too. Eric Erikson says that we humans have an innate need to leave behind a part of ourselves, a legacy if you will. Being a Dad ensures that you can pass on your wisdom (or your silliness—that's important too) in a way that it lives on after you. Being a Dad brings with it a certain pride, not only in your little soldiers who have accomplished the task but in your capacity to create a living, breathing human.

Over the years, fatherhood hasn't been much talked about because it was always considered to be okay for fathers to be just the fun parent. Today, fortunately, things are changing. Men and women are now as much equal partners in caring for the baby as making it.

Whether you have recently become a father or are preparing to be one, you are sure to have changed in some way as we made the nine-month journey through this book. I strongly believe that once you hold your baby in your arms, you will never be the same person. But as we have seen through the chapters this rewarding experience doesn't come easy. Right from financial planning to standing with your partner through her storm of symptoms, it all can be tremendously overpowering.

I often say this to anyone that will listen—mothers are superhumans that somehow just know what to do and when. And this makes sense because her womb is the only world your baby has known until very recently. The problem is, sometimes I see parents trying to turn it into a competition. What they don't realize is mothers and fathers don't necessarily play the same roles. Rather they may play complementary roles. Thus to expect that your interaction with your baby would be or should be the same as that of your partner, would be taking an overly simplistic view of the parenting dynamic.

The idea behind this book is to understand your partner's experience through these turbulent times. Pregnancies have long been misunderstood to take the spice out of a marriage. But when you as the new father understand why your partner is feeling what she is feeling and what you can do to make her feel better, it can turn into a truly rewarding experience. When partners go through an experience like this with solidarity and integrity towards each other, it gives rise to a much more cohesive unit which is exactly what the baby needs growing up.

If you enjoyed reading this book and found it helpful, please leave a review, even if it's one word like "AMAZING!". I would love to reach more fathers to help them embrace this experience with joy in their hearts, and facts in their heads. May you teach your child as much as you'll learn from them. All the very best on your new adventure, it's going to be a fun ride, I promise!

REFERENCES

Barth, L. (2020, August 19). *40 weeks pregnant: Your baby, your body, and more.* Healthline. https://www.healthline.com/health/pregnancy/40-weeks-pregnant

Ben-Joseph, E. P. (2018). *Birthing centers and hospital maternity services (for parents).* Kidshealth.org. https://kidshealth.org/en/parents/birth-centers-hospitals.html

Bradley, S. (2020, September 22). *38 weeks pregnant: Symptoms not to ignore, labor signs, more.* Healthline. https://www.healthline.com/health/pregnancy/38-weeks-pregnant

Bradley, S. (2021, September 9). *39 weeks pregnant: Symptoms, labor signs, and more.* Healthline. https://www.healthline.com/health/pregnancy/39-weeks-pregnant

Brott, A., & Ash Ruddick, J. (2021). *The expectant father.* Abbeville.

Crider, C. (2020, June 16). *Overdue baby: Causes, risks, and what you can expect.* Healthline. https://www. healthline.com/health/pregnancy/overdue-baby

Daly, K. (2014, January 1). *Love and pregnancy: 5 ways pregnancy will change your relationship.* Parents. https:// www.parents.com/pregnancy/my-life/emotions/love-and-pregnancy-5-ways-pregnancy-will-change-your-relationship/

David Gottesman. (n.d.). AZQuotes.com. Retrieved October 12, 2021, from AZQuotes.com Web site: https://www.azquotes.com/quote/535302

Donaldson-Evans, C. (2014, September 16). *1 and 2 weeks pregnant.* What to Expect; WhattoExpect. https:// www.whattoexpect.com/pregnancy/week-by-week/ weeks-1-and-2.aspx

Donaldson-Evans, C. (2021, June 24). *Week 3 of pregnancy.* What to Expect. https://www.whattoexpect. com/pregnancy/week-by-week/week-3.aspx

Grünebaum, A., McCullough, L. B., Orosz, B., & Chervenak, F. A. (2020). Neonatal mortality in the United States is related to location of birth (hospital versus home) rather than the type of birth attendant. *American*

Journal of Obstetrics and Gynecology, 223(2). https://doi.org/10.1016/j.ajog.2020.01.045

Healthline. (2017a, October 19). *4 weeks pregnant: Symptoms, tips, and more.* Healthline. https://www.healthline.com/health/pregnancy/pregnancy-week-4

Healthline. (2017b, November 3). *Low hCG levels: Causes, treatments, and symptoms.* Healthline. https://www.healthline.com/health/pregnancy/low-hcg#causes

Holland, K. (2018, September 5). *Early pregnancy symptoms.* Healthline; Healthline Media. https://www.healthline.com/health/pregnancy/early-symptoms-timeline

Holland, K. (2021, October 13). *28 weeks pregnant: Symptoms, tips, and more.* Healthline. https://www.healthline.com/health/pregnancy/28-weeks-pregnant

Horsager-Boehrer, R. (2016, March 29). *4 Tips for choosing an OB/GYN | Your pregnancy matters | UT southwestern medical center.* Utswmed.org. https://utswmed.org/medblog/choosing-obgyn/

Kay, C. (2020a, September 16). *9 weeks pregnant: Symptoms, tips, and more.* Healthline. https://www.healthline.com/health/pregnancy/pregnancy-symptoms-week-9

Kay, C. (2020b, October 1). *5 weeks pregnant: Symptoms, tips, and more.* Healthline. https://www.healthline.com/health/pregnancy/pregnancy-symptoms-week-5

Kay, C. (2020c, October 6). *10 weeks pregnant: Symptoms, tips, and more.* Healthline. https://www.healthline.com/health/pregnancy/pregnancy-symptoms-week-10

Kulp, A. (2018). *We're pregnant! : The first-time dad's pregnancy handbook.* Rockridge Press.

Marcin, A. (2017a, October 23). *20 weeks pregnancy: Symptoms, tips, and more.* Healthline. https://www.healthline.com/health/pregnancy/20-weeks-pregnant

Marcin, A. (2017b, October 23). *37 weeks pregnant: Symptoms, tips, and more.* Healthline. https://www.healthline.com/health/pregnancy/37-weeks-pregnant

McDermott, A. (2017a, October 23). *18 weeks pregnant: Symptoms, tips, and more.* Healthline. https://www.healthline.com/health/pregnancy/18-weeks-pregnant#:~:text=Symptoms%20you

McDermott, A. (2017b, October 23). *21 weeks pregnant: Symptoms, tips, and more.* Healthline. https://www.healthline.com/health/pregnancy/21-weeks-pregnant

McDermott, A. (2017c, October 23). *35 weeks pregnant: Symptoms, tips, and more.* Healthline. https://www.healthline.com/health/pregnancy/35-weeks-pregnant

Medline Plus. (2016). *Folic acid in diet: MedlinePlus medical encyclopedia.* Medlineplus.gov. https://medlineplus.gov/ency/article/002408.htm

Nemours Kids Health. (2017, June). *Diapering your baby (for parents) - Nemours Kidshealth.* Kidshealth.org. https://kidshealth.org/en/parents/diapering.html

Pevzner, H. (2021a, June 14). *Week 2 of your pregnancy.* Verywell Family. https://www.verywellfamily.com/2-weeks-pregnant-4158819

Pevzner, H. (2021b, June 14). *Week 4 of your pregnancy.* Verywell Family. https://www.verywellfamily.com/4-weeks-pregnant-4158847

Pevzner, H. P. (2021, June 14). *Week 1 of your pregnancy.* Verywell Family. https://www.verywellfamily.com/1-week-pregnant-4158813

Pfeiffer, J. (2011). *Dude, you're gonna be a dad! : How to get (both of you) through the next 9 months.* Adams Media.

Riggins Nwadike, V. (2020a, September 16). *6 weeks pregnant? Here's what to know.* Healthline. https://www.healthline.com/health/pregnancy/pregnancy-symptoms-week-6

Riggins Nwadike, V. (2020b, September 21). *7 Weeks Pregnant: Symptoms, Tips, and More.* Healthline. https://

www.healthline.com/health/pregnancy/pregnancy-symptoms-week-7

Riggins Nwadike, V. (2020c, October 6). *8 weeks pregnant: Symptoms, tips, and more.* Healthline. https://www.healthline.com/health/pregnancy/pregnancy-symptoms-week-8

Roland, J. (2017a, October 18). *29 weeks pregnant: Symptoms, tips, and more.* Healthline. https://www.healthline.com/health/pregnancy/29-weeks-pregnant

Roland, J. (2017b, October 18). *31 weeks pregnant: Symptoms, tips, and more.* Healthline. https://www.healthline.com/health/pregnancy/31-weeks-pregnant

Roland, J. (2017c, October 19). *24 weeks pregnant: Symptoms, tips, and more.* Healthline. https://www.healthline.com/health/pregnancy/24-weeks-pregnant

Roland, J. (2017d, October 23). *12 weeks pregnant: Symptoms, tips, and more.* Healthline. https://www.healthline.com/health/pregnancy/12-weeks-pregnant

Roland, J. (2017e, October 23). *16 weeks pregnant: Symptoms, tips, and more.* Healthline. https://www.healthline.com/health/pregnancy/16-weeks-pregnant

Roland, J. (2017f, October 23). *19 weeks pregnant: Symptoms, tips, and more.* Healthline. https://www.healthline.com/health/pregnancy/19-weeks-pregnant

Roland, J. (2020, October 13). *34 weeks pregnant: Symptoms, tips, and more.* Healthline. https://www.healthline.com/health/pregnancy/34-weeks-pregnant

Roland, J. (2021, August 5). *23 weeks pregnant: Symptoms, tips, and more.* Healthline. https://www.healthline.com/health/pregnancy/23-weeks-pregnant

Schaeffer, J. (2017a, October 16). *32 weeks pregnant: Symptoms, tips, and more.* Healthline. https://www.healthline.com/health/pregnancy/32-weeks-pregnant

Schaeffer, J. (2017b, October 18). *26 weeks pregnant: Symptoms, tips, and more.* Healthline. https://www.healthline.com/health/pregnancy/26-weeks-pregnant

Schaeffer, J. (2017c, October 18). *30 weeks pregnant: Symptoms, tips, and more.* Healthline. https://www.healthline.com/health/pregnancy/30-weeks-pregnant

Schaeffer, J. (2017a, October 20). *11 weeks pregnant: Symptoms, tips, and more.* Healthline. https://www.healthline.com/health/pregnancy/pregnancy-symptoms-week-11

Schaeffer, J. (2017b, October 23). *14 weeks pregnant: Symptoms, tips, and more.* Healthline. https://www.healthline.com/health/pregnancy/14-weeks-pregnant

Schaeffer, J. (2017c, October 23). *17 weeks pregnant: Symptoms, tips, and more.* Healthline. https://www.

healthline.com/health/pregnancy/17-weeks-pregnant#symptoms

Schaeffer, J. (2017d, October 23). *36 weeks pregnant: Symptoms, tips, and more*. Healthline. https://www.healthline.com/health/pregnancy/36-weeks-pregnant

Schaeffer, J. (2020, October 6). *22 weeks pregnant: Symptoms, tips, and more*. Healthline. https://www.healthline.com/health/pregnancy/22-weeks-pregnant

Silver, N. (2017a, October 18). *27 weeks pregnant: Symptoms, tips, and more*. Healthline. https://www.healthline.com/health/pregnancy/27-weeks-pregnant

Silver, N. (2017b, October 18). *33 weeks pregnant: Symptoms, tips, and more*. Healthline. https://www.healthline.com/health/pregnancy/33-weeks-pregnant

Silver, N. (2017c, October 19). *25 weeks pregnant: Symptoms, tips, and more*. Healthline. https://www.healthline.com/health/pregnancy/25-weeks-pregnant

Silver, N. (2017d, October 23). *15 weeks pregnant: Symptoms, tips, and more*. Healthline. https://www.healthline.com/health/pregnancy/15-weeks-pregnant

Wilson, D. R. (2017, August 29). *2 weeks pregnant: Symptoms, tips, and more*. Healthline. https://www.healthline.com/health/pregnancy/week-two#symptoms